DEDICATION

This book is dedicated to our patients and their families. We honor their struggle against the serious condition of schizophrenia.

ACKNOWLEDGMENT

We thank the National Alliance for Research on Schizophrenia and Depression (NARSAD), the Theodore and Vada Stanley Foundation, and the National Institutes of Health for their support of our work.

We also acknowledge and thank Shannon Mulgrew for work and support in obtaining and organizing the numerous references associated with this book. Much of the background for this work came from the teaching we have done in public hospitals and clinics throughout the country. We would like to thank the TRU and the staff in those sites for their questions and insight into our ideas.

Finally, we could not have completed this work without the support and encouragement of our families, and we thank them for their support. One of us (RRC) has been blessed with twin daughters, who send me away on my trips with the words, "We'll miss you, but we know your work is important, Dad." I would like to thank Anna and Sarah Conley for your words; they help more than you know.

Pharmacologic Treatment of Schizophrenia

First Edition

Robert R. Conley, MD
Director of the Treatment Research Unit
Maryland Psychiatric Research Center
Associate Professor of Psychiatry
and Pharmacy Practice
University of Maryland

Deanna L. Kelly, PharmD, BCPP
Maryland Psychiatric Research Center
Assistant Professor of Psychiatry
and Pharmacy Practice
University of Maryland

Professional Communications, Inc.
A Medical Publishing Company

Published by
Professional Communications, Inc.

For orders, please call
1-800-337-9838

ISBN: 1-884735-56-8

Printed in the United States of America

DISCLAIMER

The opinions expressed in this publication reflect those of the authors. However, the authors make no warranty regarding the contents of the publication. The protocols described herein are general and may not apply to a specific patient. Any product mentioned in this publication should be taken in accordance with the prescribing information provided by the manufacturer.

This text is printed on recycled paper.

Table of Contents

TABLES

FIGURES

Introduction

There have been many "revolutions" in the care and treatment of people with schizophrenia over the past century. The most promising was the introduction of specific antipsychotic medications in the 1950s and 1960s. These medications, along with a marked societal change in the way the mentally ill are treated (with an emphasis on community as opposed to institutional treatment), have improved the life of most people who suffer from schizophrenia. The goal of normal functioning, however, remains elusive for most people with this illness. Unemployment, inadequate housing, and a high death rate continue to be common problems for these people. One of the major reasons for this has been that traditional antipsychotic medications, while helpful in controlling some of the obvious symptoms of schizophrenia, do not control all of the symptoms of this illness and are associated with serious lifestyle-limiting side effects.

In the 1990s, a new group of medications was introduced. These drugs are more effective and have fewer side effects than traditional medications. However, they are not a cure and have serious side effects of their own. Furthermore, people who take these medications are generally much more capable of experiencing and showing emotions than people who take traditional medications. This helps people to live better but makes them appear much less controlled than people who take traditional medications. For this reason, clinicians must use new outcome measures to judge the effectiveness of a medication.

We hope this book helps clinicians in their search for the appropriate medication regimen for each of their patients. We need to be careful about claims that the new medications represent another revolution. We do feel, however, that most people who suffer from schizophrenia today can lead a much better life with the optimal use of the second-generation antipsychotics.

This book has been prepared for clinicians as a review of the treatment and management of schizophrenia and other serious chronic psychotic disorders. The authors would like to thank the clinicians and investigators whose observations and publications have added to our own work in this exciting area. Their contributions have made this timely presentation of new pharmacotherapies for schizophrenia possible.

1 General Information About Schizophrenia

1

Epidemiology

Schizophrenia is one of the more challenging and complex psychiatric disorders that afflict humans. The core symptoms of this illness are highly variable among patients, with a wide array of symptoms such as:

- Hallucinations
- Delusions
- Disorganized speech and behavior
- Inappropriate affect
- Cognitive deficits
- Impaired psychosocial functioning.

The onset of symptoms in most cases is insidious, usually preceded by a prodromal phase characterized by:

- Gradual social withdrawal
- Diminished interests
- Changes in appearance and hygiene
- Changes in cognition
- Bizarre or odd behavior.

Descriptions of chronic severe functional psychosis date back as far as human literature. Often psychotic symptoms were considered to be signs or manifestations of supernatural influences on the individual. Psychotic individuals have held the burden of being shunned and feared by society in general. Greek physicians first wrote about the concept that mental illness was due to natural forces (eg, a disease). This concept was not embraced by Western physicians until the Renaissance but was kept alive by Arabic physicians who practiced classical medicine. During the 17th and 18th centuries, the first Western mental hospitals were established and much work went into characterizing and describing mental illness. Morel, in 1860, first proposed the term "deménce précoce" to describe a progressive insanity in the young. Kraepelin, in 1896, building on this work and that of others, such as Hecker and Kahlbaum, distinguished "dementia praecox" from manic-depressive psychosis. Kraepelin believed that this condition always progressed to marked dementia. In 1911, Eugene Bleuler coined the term schizophrenia, defining a disorder that included dementia praecox but also other forms of progressive psychosis that did not deteriorate as severely. This work gave rise to our modern concept of schizophrenia (Table 1.1). As we better understand the brain and central nervous system (CNS) pathophysiology, diagnosis and treatment will continue to change.

TABLE 1.1— SUMMARY OF EPIDEMIOLOGIC FACTORS
Lifetime Prevalence • 1% in both males and females • Occurs in most areas of the world
Onset of Illness • Late adolescence/early adulthood • Earlier in males
Average Age at First Hospitalization • Males—15 to 24 years • Females—25 to 34 years

Pathophysiology

1

Advances in technology have provided a means for investigating functional and structural abnormalities in the brain through the use of:

- Positron emission tomography (PET)
- Single photon emission computed tomography (SPECT)
- Functional magnetic resonance imaging (fMRI).

This technology has led to advancement in the field of schizophrenia research in determining areas of disturbance in certain brain regions (Table 1.2). Unfortunately, however, research in this area has not yet led to the identification of the basic neuropathology of the disorder.

TABLE 1.2 — SUMMARY OF STRUCTURAL AND FUNCTIONAL ABNORMALITIES
• Cortical atrophy (prefrontal lobe, medial temporal cortex) • Diencephalic gliosis (hippocampus, amygdala) • Ventricular dilation (particularly left sided) • Cerebellar atrophy (vermis) • Reversal of normal frontal and occipital lobe asymmetries

Functional changes in the brain of people with schizophrenia are highly correlated with certain symptoms. Therefore functional imaging has progressed along the lines of delineating the metabolic changes associated with specific symptom complexes. Positive symptoms, negative symptoms, and cognitive disturbances, all more fully described later in this chapter, are associated with specific functional changes in the brain (Table 1.3).

TABLE 1.3 — SPECIFIC FUNCTIONAL CHANGES IN THE BRAIN		
Symptom Complex	**Brain Region**	**↑/↓ in Activity***
Thought disorder	Anterior cingulate gyrus	↑
Reality distortions/ delusions	Left prefrontal cortex	↓
Positive symptoms	Left hippocampus	↑
Auditory hallucinations	Broca's area, superior temporal cortex	↑
Negative symptoms	Left prefrontal cortex	↓
Psychomotor poverty	Inferior parietal cortex	↓
Anhedonia	Right inferior parietal cortex, cingulate gyrus	↑
* Compared with normal controls.		

The introduction of effective antipsychotic medications in the mid-1950s opened the door for studies assessing neurochemical hypotheses of schizophrenia. The advent of highly sensitive assays that measure CNS neurotransmitter levels, their metabolites, and related metabolic enzymes prompted the development of hypotheses proposing that neurotransmitters have a role in the causation of schizophrenia.

The most common pathophysiologic theories associated with the etiology of schizophrenia involve the dopaminergic system. This hypothesis began in the late 1950s when it was discovered that antipsychotic drugs are postsynaptic dopamine antagonists. It has been observed that drugs that increase dopamine will enhance or produce positive psychotic symptoms (cocaine, amphetamines) and drugs such as antipsychotics that decrease dopamine will decrease or stop positive symptoms. There are four dopamine tracts of primary interest in the brain (Figure 1.1). A basic knowledge of these tracts and their relationship is important for understanding the therapeutic and adverse effects of both traditional and second-generation antipsychotic drugs (SGADs) (Table 1.4).

FIGURE 1.1 — PRINCIPAL DOPAMINE PATHWAYS IN THE BRAIN

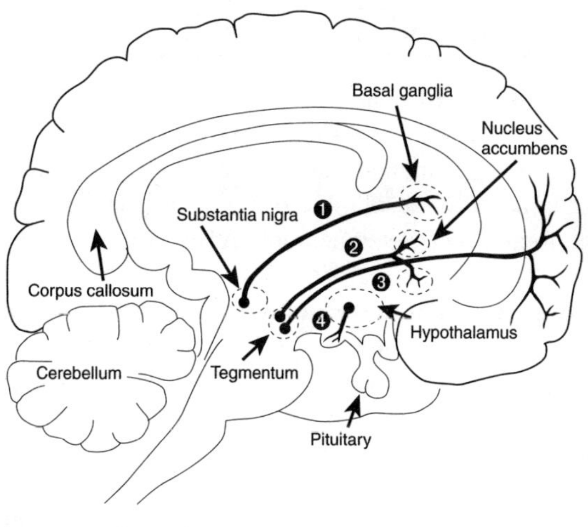

(1) The nigrostriatal tract, also known as the extrapyramidal pathway, begins in the substantia nigra and ends in the caudate nucleus and putamen of the basal ganglia. (2) The mesolimbic tract originates in the midbrain tegmentum and innervates the nucleus accumbens and adjacent limbic structures. (3) The mesocortical tract originates in the midbrain tegmentum and innervates anterior cortical areas. (4) The tuberoinfundibular tract projects from the arcuate and periventricular nuclei of the hypothalamus to the intermediate lobe of the pituitary and to the portal blood system surrounding the anterior pituitary.

Martin MB, et al. In: *Textbook of Neuropsychiatry*. Washington, DC: American Psychiatric Press; 1997:55-85.

TABLE 1.4 — SUMMARY OF DOPAMINE TRACTS AND EFFECTS OF ANTIPSYCHOTICS	
Dopamine Tract	**Effect of Antipsychotic**
Nigrostriatal	Movement disorder
Mesolimbic	Relief of psychosis
Mesocortical	Increase in negative symptoms, akathisia?
Tuberoinfundibular	Increased prolactin concentrations

The nigrostriatal tract originates in the A9 area of the substantia nigra and terminates with the synapses in the putamen and caudate nucleus of the basal ganglia. The mesolimbic pathway projects from the midbrain ventral tegmentum (A10) to the cingulate gyrus and limbic regions. The mesocortical tract extends from A10 to the prefrontal and frontal cortex. The tuberoinfundibular tract originates in the hypothalamus and projects to the pituitary gland.

There is much evidence supporting the dopaminergic receptor deficit hypothesis. Increased glucose metabolism in the basal ganglia and decreased metabolism in the frontal cortex may be indicative of dopaminergic hyperactivity and hypoactivity in these regions, respectively. PET studies measuring receptor densities using dopamine $(D)_2$-specific ligands such as raclopride show increased densities of D_2 receptors in the basal ganglia and decreased densities in the prefrontal cortex. Other direct evidence supporting the validity of the dopamine hypothesis comes from postmortem evaluation of tissues and plasma. Investigators have measured the amount of dopamine and its metabolites, such as homovanillic acid (HVA). The brain of people with schizophrenia has increased presynaptic dopamine and/or HVA levels in areas of the mesocortical and mesolimbic systems as compared with that of normal controls.

The hypothesis that the dopamine system explains schizophrenia symptoms is far from complete. Recently, it has been suggested that combined dysfunction of the dopamine and glutamate transmitter systems may better explain this disorder. Phencyclidine (PCP) and ketamine are psychotomimetic drugs which noncompetitively block the ion channel of the glutamate subtype receptor, the *N*-methyl-D-aspartate (NMDA) receptor. These agents can elicit the full range of psychotic symptoms resembling those of schizophrenia. Based on this model of schizophrenia, NMDA receptor hypofunction, as a type of transmitter disturbance, may explain many of the symptoms seen in this illness. Dopamine transmission is intrinsically tied to glutamate release and may explain why medications that antagonize dopamine may partially work in this disorder. Dopamine receptors may inhibit glutamate release; thus a defect in the dopamine system that causes hyperactivity could result in excessive suppression of glutamate release at NMDA receptors. The net effect would be hypofunction of the NMDA receptor system as the basis for schizophrenic symptoms.

There has also been a great deal of speculation regarding the role of serotonin receptor antagonism in regard to antipsychotic effects. Many traditional antipsychotics are highly active at serotonin receptors, but this property does not distinguish the clinical effects of these drugs in a meaningful way. The serotonin hypothesis of psychosis actually predates the dopamine hypothesis, largely because of lysergic acid diethylamide (LSD), a drug with psychotomimetic properties that releases serotonin. Interest in this theory was rekindled by the finding that clozapine, which has a 100-fold selectivity for serotonin compared with dopamine receptors, is highly efficacious. The other SGADs also have high serotonin-to-dopamine binding ratios. Serotonin receptor binding may be important to these drugs' actions, possibly by stimulating dopamine activity in mesocortical pathways. However, a compelling theory relating dopamine and serotonin receptor affinities has not yet been developed.

Genetic Predisposition

There may be a lesion present at birth with the potential for NMDA receptor hypofunction, and this may not trigger psychopathologic or neuropathologic processes until late adolescence, at which time it would begin to trigger schizophrenic symptoms. There is fairly strong evidence that schizophrenia is at least partially genetic in nature. The risks are listed in Table 1.5.

TABLE 1.5 — RISK OF DEVELOPING SCHIZOPHRENIA

Risk Factor	Risk (%)
First-degree relative is diagnosed	10
Both parents are diagnosed	40
Dizygotic twins	10
Monozygotic twins	40 to 50

Many genes have been weakly associated with the development of schizophrenia. However, there is probably no single "schizophrenic gene." The possible genetic effect is a susceptibility to schizophrenia, with either a certain gene or a combination of several genes necessary for development of the disorder (Table 1.6).

TABLE 1.6 — GENES IDENTIFIED AS SCHIZOPHRENIA RELATED	
Amount of Evidence	**Genes**
Significant evidence	13, 22
Weak evidence	6, 8, 10, 14, 15

Clinical Presentation

Schizophrenia is a chronic disorder of thought, affect, and a significant disturbance in the individual's ability to function in society and develop interpersonal relationships. The clinical presentation of this disorder can be extremely varied, and despite the attempts to portray a stereotype in the media, the stereotypic schizophrenic individual does not exist. The categorization of independent pathophysiologic processes underlying signs and symptoms dates back to Kraepelin. He proposed that there were two processes characterizing schizophrenia. The first domain was a "weakening of those emotional activities which permanently form the mainsprings of volition." "Emotional dullness, loss of volition, and failure of mental activities" were the results of this domain and termed the "avolitional syndrome." This was the predecessor of the current concept of primary negative symptoms or the deficit syndrome. Kraepelin's second domain "consisted in the loss of the inner unity of the activities of intellect, emotion, and volition, in themselves and one another."

In the 1970s, Strauss and others suggested that schizophrenic symptoms fall into three specific symptom complexes: positive symptoms, negative symptoms, and disorders of relating. Carpenter and others further characterized these three symptom domains into psychotic disturbances, cognitive dysfunction, and negative symptoms.

■ Psychotic Symptoms

The acute psychotic symptoms include:

- Hallucinations (distortion or exaggeration of perception)
- Delusions (fixed false beliefs).

Hallucinations may occur as auditory, visual, olfactory, gustatory, and tactile, but auditory hallucinations are the most common type in patients with schizophrenia. Voices frequently occur and are distinct from the person's own thoughts. The content of hallucinations is variable but is often threatening or commanding. Delusions are erroneous beliefs that usually involve a misinterpretation of perceptions or experiences. Types of delusions are listed in Table 1.7.

■ Cognitive Symptoms

Subtle disturbance in associative thinking may develop years before disorganized thinking (formal thought disorder). Inferences about thought are based primarily on the individual's speech. Thinking and speech of patients are frequently incomprehensible to others and often are illogical. Characteristics of formal thought disorder are listed in Table 1.8.

■ Negative Symptoms

Primary negative symptoms or deficit symptoms are quite ubiquitous in schizophrenia; however, they are difficult to evaluate because they occur in a continuum with normality, are nonspecific, and are often due to medication side effects (secondary negative symptoms), mood disorder, environmental understimulation, or demoralization. The best test for establishing true negative symptoms is to examine their persistence for a considerable period of time despite efforts directed at resolving the other causes. Approximately 10% to 15% of schizophrenics may exhibit the

TABLE 1.7 — TYPES OF DELUSIONS	
Delusion	**Description**
Ideas of reference	Conviction that there are "meanings" behind events, media, and people's actions that are directed specifically toward oneself
Delusions of influence	Belief that one can control events through telepathy or other means
Persecutory delusions	Belief that one is being tormented, followed, tricked, spied on, or subjected to ridicule
Thought broadcasting	Belief that others can hear or read one's thoughts
Thought insertion	Belief that someone else's thoughts have been inserted into one's mind
Bizarre delusions	Belief involving a phenomenon that the person's culture would regard as totally implausible
Grandiose delusions	Feelings of inflated worth, power, talents, knowledge, identity, importance, or special relationship with famous people or a deity
Somatic delusions	Belief concerning the appearance or functioning of one's body
Ergotomatic delusions	Belief that another person, usually of higher status, is in love with one
Derealization	Perception of the world as unreal
Depersonalization	Feeling of removal from the reality of one's body
Lack of insight	Unawareness of illness or need for treatment even though it is evident to others

TABLE 1.8 — CHARACTERISTICS OF FORMAL THOUGHT DISORDER	
Loosening of associations	Disconnected ideas and jumping from topic to unconnected topic
Neologisms	Coining new words (may have symbolic meaning)
Tangentiality	Abandoning one's ideational objective in pursuit of thoughts peripheral to the original goal
Word salad	Displaying an incomprehensible mixture of words and phrases
Overinclusiveness	Disruption of the flow of thoughts by inclusion of irrelevant information
Thought blocking	Halting of speech, often in mid-sentence, which is then picked up later, usually at another point in the thought process
Clanging	Selection of words and themes based on the sound of the words used rather than on thought content
Echolalia	Repetition of words or phrases in a musical or sing-song fashion but without an apparent effort to communicate
Concreteness	Poor ability to think in abstract terms, despite normal or above average intelligence quotient (IQ)
Circumstantiality	Giving an extensive description of insignificant detail before eventually arriving at the original goal
Perseveration	Repeating a response to varied stimuli

majority of psychopathology as negative symptoms. Such patients may be referred to as having a "deficit syndrome" (Table 1.9).

1

TABLE 1.9 — NEGATIVE SYMPTOMS	
Symptoms	**Description**
Alogia	Speaking very little but without being intentionally resistant (poverty of speech) or may speak a normal amount but say very little (poverty of speech content)
Anhedonia	Loss of joy and interest in activities
Avolition	Inability to initiate and persist in goal-directed activities; may prevent one from completing activities
Blunted affect	Facial appearance that is immobile and unresponsive, with poor eye contact and reduced body language
Poor social skills	Diminished social involvement associated with unwarranted fear, hostility, distrust, apathy, or passivity
Poor grooming	Neglect and apathy concerning appearance and hygiene

■ Presentation of Symptoms

Patients with schizophrenia may be uncooperative, hostile, and verbally or physically aggressive due to their misinterpretation of reality and often due to command hallucinations. Difficulty with anxiety may be exhibited due to positive symptoms and suspiciousness. Patients may have impaired self-care skills and may be dirty and unkempt due to negative symptoms. Sleep and appetite are often disturbed. Patients often have difficulty living independently in the community and have difficulty forming close relationships with others. Additionally, such patients have problems with initiating or maintaining employment and are often noncompliant with medications, thereby increasing their risk for relapse.

Diagnosis

The commonly accepted diagnostic criteria for schizophrenia come from the *Diagnostic and Statistical Manual of Mental Disorders*, 4th edition (DSM-IV). The essential features are a mixture of characteristic signs and symptoms as listed above that have been present for a significant portion of time during a 1-month period (or a shorter time if successfully treated), with some signs of the disorder persisting for at least 6 months. These signs and symptoms are:

- Associated with marked social or occupational dysfunction
- Not accounted for by a mood disorder
- Not due to the direct physiologic effects of a substance or a general medical condition (Table 1.10)

There are subtypes of schizophrenia that are defined by predominant symptomatology at the time of evaluation. The clinical picture present at the most recent evaluation or admission is the subtype usually given to categorize the patient and may, therefore, change over time. Not infrequently, the presentation may include symptoms that are characteristic of more than one subtype. The subtypes are assigned according to the following categories:

- *Catatonic type* is whenever prominent catatonic symptoms are present (regardless of the presence of other symptoms).
- *Disorganized type* is assigned whenever disorganization of speech and behavior and flat or inappropriate affect are prominent.

- *Paranoid type* is assigned whenever there is a preoccupation with delusions or frequent hallucinations.
- *Undifferentiated type* is a category describing presentations that include prominent active-phase symptoms not meeting other types.
- *Residual type* is assigned to presentations in which there is continuing evidence of the disturbance, but the criteria for the active-phase symptoms are no longer met.

Differential diagnosis of psychotic signs and symptoms is shown in Table 1.11.

Course and Prognosis

Although the course of schizophrenia is variable, the long-term prognosis for independent function is often poor. This illness is marked by intermittent acute psychotic episodes and a downward decline in psychosocial functioning. A patient may become more withdrawn, bizarre, and nonfunctional over many years. Complete return to full premorbid functioning is not common in this disorder. Many of the more dramatic and acute symptoms will disappear with time, but severe residual symptoms may persist. Family and friends may find this illness difficult to interpret and understand. Involvement with the law is fairly common for misdemeanors such as vagrancy, loitering, and disturbing the peace. The overall life expectancy is shortened primarily due to suicide, accidents, and the inability for self-care. The lifetime risk of suicide for patients with schizophrenia is 10% to 13%, with an incidence of 350 to 600/100,000 compared with 11/100,000 in the general population. Patients who have fewer periods of acute psychotic episodes and those who are treated early in their course of illness may have a better prognosis. Persistent compliance with

TABLE 1.10 — DIAGNOSTIC CRITERIA FOR SCHIZOPHRENIA

A. *Characteristic Symptoms:* Two (or more) of the following, each present for a significant portion of time during a 1-month period (or less if successfully treated):
   (1) Delusions
   (2) Hallucinations
   (3) Disorganized speech (eg, frequent derailment or incoherence)
   (4) Grossly disorganized or catatonic behavior
   (5) Negative symptoms, ie, affective flattening, alogia, or avolition

   NOTE: Only one Criterion A symptom is required if delusions are bizarre or hallucinations consist of a voice keeping up a running commentary on the person's behavior or thoughts, or two or more voices conversing with each other.

B. *Social/Occupational Dysfunction:* For a significant portion of the time since the onset of the disturbance, one or more major areas of functioning such as work, interpersonal relations, or self-care are markedly below the level achieved prior to the onset (or when the onset is in childhood or adolescence, failure to achieve expected level of interpersonal, academic, or occupational achievement).

C. *Duration:* Continuous signs of the disturbance persist for at least 6 months. This 6-month period must include at least 1 month of symptoms (or less if successfully treated) that meet Criterion A (ie, active-phase symptoms) and may include periods of prodromal or residual symptoms. During these prodromal or residual periods, the signs of the disturbance may be manifested by only negative symptoms or two or more symptoms listed in Criterion A present in an attenuated form (eg, odd beliefs, unusual perceptual experiences).

D. *Schizoaffective and Mood Disorder Exclusion:* Schizoaffective disorder and mood disorder with psychotic features have been ruled out because either:
(1) No major depressive, manic, or mixed episodes have occurred concurrently with the active-phase symptoms; or
(2) If mood episodes have occurred during active phase symptoms, their total duration has been brief relative to the duration of the active and residual periods.

E. *Substance/General Medical Condition Exclusion:* The disturbance is not due to the direct physiological effects of a substance (eg, a drug of abuse, a medication) or a general medical condition.

F. *Relationship to a Pervasive Developmental Disorder:* If there is a history of autistic disorder or another pervasive developmental disorder, the additional diagnosis of schizophrenia is made only if prominent delusions or hallucinations are also present for at least 1 month (or less if successfully treated).

Classification of longitudinal course (can be applied only after at least 1 year has elapsed since the initial onset of active-phase symptoms):

- *Episodic With Interepisode Residual Symptoms* (episodes are defined by the reemergence of prominent psychotic symptoms); also specify if: *With Prominent Negative Symptoms*
- *Episodic With No Interepisode Residual Symptoms*
- *Continuous* (prominent psychotic symptoms are present throughout the period of observation); also specify if: *With Prominent Negative Symptoms*
- *Single Episode in Partial Remission*; also specify if: *With Prominent Negative Symptoms*
- *Single Episode in Full Remission*
- *Other or Unspecified Pattern*

American Psychiatric Association. *Diagnostic and Statistical Manual of Mental Disorders*. 4th ed. Washington, DC: American Psychiatric Press; 1994.

TABLE 1.11 — DIFFERENTIAL DIAGNOSIS OF PSYCHOTIC SIGNS AND SYMPTOMS
• Schizoaffective disorder • Mood disorder • Dementia • Delirium • Drug intoxication • Pervasive developmental disorder • Neurologic conditions (neoplasms, migraines, Huntington's chorea, deafness, epilepsy) • Metabolic conditions (hypoxia, hypercapnia, hypoglycemia) • Endocrine conditions (hyperthyroidism, hypothyroidism, hyperparathyroidism, hypoparathyroidism, hypoadrenocorticism) • Fluid or electrolyte imbalances • Hepatic or renal disease • Autoimmune disorders • Hypnagogic and hypnopompic hallucinations

a tolerable drug regimen also improves prognosis (Table 1.12). Some symptoms will respond better to treatment than others (Figure 1.2).

The natural history of antipsychotic-treated schizophrenia is poorly understood, since traditional antipsychotics tended to cause many side effects that

TABLE 1.12 — CLINICAL CHARACTERISTICS ASSOCIATED WITH AN IMPROVED PROGNOSIS
• No family history of schizophrenia • Rapid onset of active psychotic symptoms • Good premorbid social and occupational functioning • Probable precipitating stress to the acute psychosis • No evidence of central nervous system abnormalities • Marriage • Paranoid subtype • Later onset of illness • Early temporal treatment in the course of illness

FIGURE 1.2 — RESPONSIVENESS OF SYMPTOMS

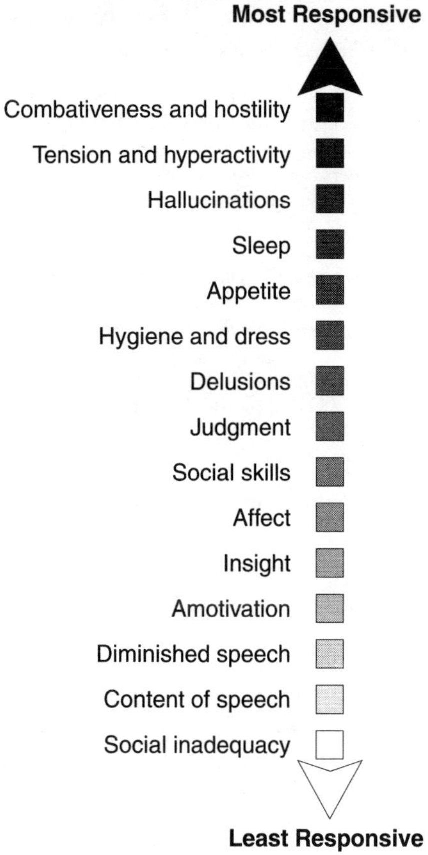

markedly lessened compliance and increased the incidence of negative symptoms in chronic patients. It remains to be seen whether the SGADs will offer better outcomes in the long term; however, based on their first 5 years of use in the clinical setting, there is much cause for hope. The order of responsiveness of symptoms may change as the number of patients treated with SGADs increases.

SUGGESTED READING

American Psychiatric Association. *Diagnostic and Statistical Manual of Mental Disorders*. 4th ed. (DSM-IV). Washington, DC: American Psychiatric Press, Inc; 1994.

Andreasen NC, Carpenter WT Jr. Diagnosis and classification of schizophrenia. *Schizophr Bull*. 1993;19:199-214.

Carlsson A, Waters N, Carlsson ML. Neurotransmitter interactions in schizophrenia—therapeutic implications. *Biol Psychiatry*. 1999; 46:1388-1395.

Farber NB, Newcomer JW, Olney JW. The glutamate synapse in neuropsychiatric disorders. Focus on schizophrenia and Alzheimer's disease. *Prog Brain Res*. 1998;116:421-437.

Gelman S. *Medicating Schizophrenia: A History*. New Brunswick, NJ and London, UK: Rutgers University Press; 1999.

Martin MB, Owen CM, Morihisa JM. An overview of neurotransmitters and neuroceptors. In: Hales RE, Yudofsky SC, eds. *Textbook of Neuropsychiatry*. Washington DC: American Psychiatric Press; 1997:55-85.

McClure RJ, Keshavan MS, Pettegrew JW. Chemical and physiologic brain imaging in schizophrenia. *Psychiatr Clin North Am*. 1998;21:93-122.

Pearlson GD, Marsh L. Structural brain imaging in schizophrenia: a selective review. *Biol Psychiatry*. 1999;46:627-649.

Tsuang MT, Stone WS, Faraone SV. Schizophrenia: a review of genetic studies. *Harv Rev Psychiatry*. 1999;7:185-207.

2 Treatment of Schizophrenia

2

History

Antipsychotic drugs are used to treat nearly all forms of psychosis, including:

- Schizophrenia
- Schizoaffective disorder
- Affective disorders with psychosis
- Dementias.

The first antipsychotic drugs available, the traditional or conventional antipsychotics as termed in this book, were previously referred to as neuroleptic agents. These drugs all have important limitations to their use:

- They are not effective in all patients.
- They have several serious adverse effects.
- They have a history of poor long-term outcomes associated with their use.

These limitations have prompted a search for newer medications with better side effect profiles and improved effectiveness.

Chlorpromazine was the first conventional antipsychotic available. This drug was first developed for controlling preoperative anxiety, but within its first year of use it was recognized as a potential treatment for psychosis. This medication gained rapid acceptance due to the lack of other effective treatments for psychosis. Many other medications, such as thioridazine, fluphenazine, haloperidol, and thiothixene, were marketed shortly thereafter. The second-generation antipsychotic drugs (SGADs) (atypical or novel antipsychotics) were first introduced in the late 1980s, with the prototypical agent, clozapine. This class of medication differed primarily by producing minimal or no extrapyramidal symptoms in humans and catalepsy (defined as immobility for 20 seconds) in rodents. These agents treat a broader spectrum of symptoms of schizophrenia as compared with traditional agents.

Available Antipsychotic Drugs

This chapter will cover the available antipsychotic medications and their place in therapy. Chapter 3, *Second-Generation Antipsychotic Drugs,* and Chapter 4, *Conventional Antipsychotic Drugs,* will cover each class of medication more thoroughly. The available antipsychotics are listed in Table 2.1. More specific details on dosing and available preparations are located in the next chapters.

Treatment Recommendations

Traditional antipsychotics were considered the gold standard for treatment prior to the advent of novel antipsychotics. Despite their numerous advantages, however, the SGADs have not routinely moved into first-line therapy for all patients. This primarily has been due to two reasons:

- Novel agents lack the neuroleptic or tranquilizing effect that many clinicians were accustomed to and relied upon for initial therapy.
- The cost of newer medications is higher than the cost of traditional agents.

In 1999, traditional antipsychotic drugs accounted for about 36% of all agents being used in the United States. Twenty-seven percent of patients were on risperidone; 22%, olanzapine; 7%, quetiapine; and 8%, clozapine. Over the past several years, the number of patients on traditional agents has dropped from about 60% to 40%, while the use of SGADs has been increasing. Clinicians are realizing the benefits of atypical drugs as compared with traditional antipsychotics and are utilizing benzodiazepines and other strategies for acute treatment and agitation (see Chapter 6, *Management of Acute Psychosis, Psychiatric Emergencies, and Aggressive/Suicidal Behavior*). Additionally, accumulating evidence suggests that despite the higher cost of SGADs, these medications are more cost-effective than traditional agents (see Chapter 12, *Outcomes and Health-Services Research*). Thus SGADs (not including clozapine) are now considered to be first-line therapy for most patients with schizophrenia.

Treatment recommendations have been developed through the use of consensus guidelines and algorithms. Some medication recommendations from the Schizophrenia Patient Outcomes Research Team project are listed in Table 2.2.

The most recent set of treatment guidelines comes from the Expert Consensus Guidelines for the Treatment of Schizophrenia, which was published by the *Journal of Clinical Psychiatry* in 1999. These guidelines are based on information from leaders in the field of psychiatric research concerning standards of practice for the treatment of schizophrenia. Table 2.3 lists recommendations for antipsychotic use in certain situations.

Rating Scales

Unlike many other branches of medicine, psychiatry—and specifically the treatment of schizophrenia—lacks laboratory or other biologic measures that can be used to assess the presence, severity, or response to treatment. Objective rating scales to assess a wide variety of symptoms and side effects exist to help both the clinician and the researcher determine how a pa-

TABLE 2.1 — AVAILABLE ANTIPSYCHOTIC DRUGS FOR THE TREATMENT OF SCHIZOPHRENIA

Generic Name	Trade Name	Manufacturer	Conventional Equivalent Dose (mg)
Conventional Antipsychotic Drugs			
Chlorpromazine	Thorazine, others	SmithKline Beecham	100
Fluphenazine	Many	Many	2
Haloperidol	Haldol	Ortho-McNeil	2
Loxapine	Loxitane	Watson	10
Mesoridazine	Serentil	Boehringer Ingelheim	50
Molindone	Moban	Endo	10
Perphenazine	Trilafon	Schering	10
Pimozide	Orap	Gate	1
Thioridazine	Many	Mylan, others	100
Thiothixene	Navane	Pfizer	4
Trifluoperazine	Stelazine, others	SmithKline Beecham, others	5

Second-Generation Antipsychotic Drugs			
Clozapine	Clozaril	Novartis	50*
Olanzapine	Zyprexa	Lilly	10*
Quetiapine	Seroquel	AstraZeneca	50*
Risperidone	Risperdal	Janssen	1*

* Second-generation antipsychotic drugs, unlike conventional agents, do not have clinical dose ranges that can be easily predicted from *in vitro* activity. The "dose equivalents" given here are approximate and based on clinical observations.

TABLE 2.2 — SCHIZOPHRENIA TREATMENT RECOMMENDATIONS

- Antipsychotic medications other than clozapine should be used as the first-line treatment to reduce psychotic symptoms in persons experiencing an acute-symptom episode of schizophrenia.
- The dosage of antipsychotic medication for an acute-symptom episode should be in the range of 300 to 1,000 chlorpromazine (CPZ) equivalents per day for a minimum of 6 weeks.* Reasons for dosages outside this range should be justified and the minimal effective dose should be used.
- Prophylactic use of antiparkinsonian agents to reduce the incidence of extrapyramidal symptoms (EPS) should be determined on a case-by-case basis, taking into account patient and physician preferences, prior individual history of EPS, and other risk factors for both EPS and anticholinergic side effects. The effectiveness of and continued need for antiparkinsonian agents should be assessed in an ongoing fashion.
- Persons who experience acute-symptom relief with an antipsychotic medication should continue to receive this medication for at least 1 year subsequent to symptom stabilization to reduce the risk of relapse or worsening of positive symptoms.
- The maintenance dosage of antipsychotic medication should be in the range of 300 to 600 CPZ equivalents (oral or depot) per day.*
- Depot antipsychotic maintenance therapy should be strongly considered in persons who have difficulty complying with an oral medication regimen or who prefer the depot regimen.
- Persons who experience persistent and clinically significant associated symptoms of anxiety, depression, or hostility, despite an adequate reduction in positive symptoms with antipsychotic therapy, should receive a trial of adjunctive pharmacotherapy.

• Persons who experience persistent and clinically significant positive symptoms despite adequate antipsychotic therapy, including trials with newer antipsychotics, should receive a trial of adjunctive pharmacotherapy.
* This dosage range was based on the use of conventional antipsychotics and cannot be exactly translated into an appropriate dosage for second-generation antipsychotic drugs.
Lehman AF, Steinwachs DM. *Schizophr Bull.* 1998;24:11-20.

tient is doing. Several rating scales are used in assessing the treatment of schizophrenia.

Efficacy Measures

■ Brief Psychiatric Rating Scale

The Brief Psychiatric Rating Scale is an 18-item scale that measures major symptoms, both psychotic and nonpsychotic (Figure 2.1). It is appropriate for assessing baseline psychopathology, clinical course, and treatment response. This instrument is rated on a 7-point scale (1 = not present, 7 = extremely severe). This scale is probably the most widely used scale in the assessment of schizophrenia treatment and has been found to be reliable. A 20% decrease in symptoms is often used as a standard of response on this rating scale.

■ Clinical Global Impression

The Clinical Global Impression is a 3-item scale that assesses treatment response in psychiatric patients. It is used to monitor clinical course and may be administered to many diagnostic groups of patients. The three items include:

- Severity of illness
- Global improvement
- Efficacy index.

TABLE 2.3 — RECOMMENDATIONS FOR ANTIPSYCHOTIC USE IN CERTAIN SITUATIONS

- First-episode schizophrenic patients with predominately positive symptoms should be treated with second-generation antipsychotic drugs (SGADs) as first-line therapy.
- The recommended antipsychotics for persistent aggression and violence are clozapine and high-potency traditional agents.
- Recommended antipsychotics in patients with insomnia include SGADs and low-potency traditional agents.
- SGADs are preferred over conventional agents in patients with:
  - Comorbid substance abuse
  - Dysphoria
  - Cognitive problems.
- Clozapine is the preferred agent in patients who exhibit excessive water drinking.
- Risperidone or ziprasidone* is preferred in patients when sedation should be avoided.
- Risperidone, quetiapine, or ziprasidone* is preferred in patients when weight gain should be avoided.
- SGADs should be used in patients when extrapyramidal symptoms should be avoided.
- Risperidone, ziprasidone*, quetiapine, and high-potency agents should be used in patients when anticholinergic effects should be avoided.
- Ziprasidone*, quetiapine, olanzapine, or clozapine should be used in patients when sexual/reproductive side effects should be avoided.

* Investigational.

Item 1 is rated on a seven-point scale (1 = normal, 7 among the most extremely ill patients) as is item 2 (1 = very much improved, 7 = very much worse). Item 3 is rated on a 4-point scale (from "none" to "outweighs therapeutic effects"). The brevity of the scale, its simplicity, and its high validity are all favorable aspects of this scale. This scale is easily used in routine clinical care.

■ Positive and Negative Syndrome Scale

The Positive and Negative Syndrome Scale (PANSS) is a 30-item rating scale that assesses positive, negative, and other symptoms in patients with schizophrenia. The instrument is rated on a 7-point scale (1 = absent, 7 = extreme). Seven items each are grouped to form a positive scale and a negative scale. High inter-rater reliability and test-retest reliability have been demonstrated for the scale. Additionally, the PANSS shows a close correspondence with the Scale for the Assessment of Negative Symptoms and the Scale for the Assessment of Positive Symptoms.

■ Global Assessment Scale

The Global Assessment Scale (GAS) is a single-item rating scale for evaluating overall functioning of a subject during a specified period (Figure 2.2). The period assessed is usually the week prior to administration. The scoring ranges from 1 to 100, with 100 being the healthiest individual to 1, the most ill. The Global Assessment of Functioning (GAF) scale, which is used for rating Axis V of the *Diagnostic and Statistical Manual of Mental Disorders*, 4th edition is a revision of the GAS. The GAF has slightly differing anchor points and does not include individuals with superior functioning. A score on the GAF equates to normal functioning with no symptoms.

Side Effect Scales

The three most widely used rating instruments for side effects in patients treated with antipsychotics include:

- Simpson-Angus Scale (SAS)

FIGURE 2.1 — BRIEF PSYCHIATRIC RATING SCALE

Subject ______________________

Rater ______________________

Date ______________________

	Not Present	Very Mild	Mild	Moderate	Moderate-Severe	Severe	Very Severe	Not Assessed
1. *Somatic Concern*—Degree of concern over present bodily health. Rate the degree to which physical health is perceived as a problem by the patient, whether complaints have a realistic basis or not.	1	2	3	4	5	6	7	8
2. *Anxiety*—Worry, fear, or overconcern for present or future. Rate solely on the basis of verbal report of patient's own subjective experiences. Do not infer anxiety from physical signs of neurotic defense mechanisms.	1	2	3	4	5	6	7	8
3. *Emotional Withdrawal*—Deficiency in relating to the interviewer and to the interview situation. Rate only the degree to which the patient gives the impression of failing to be in emotional contact with other people in the interview situation.	1	2	3	4	5	6	7	8
4. *Conceptual Disorganization*—Degree to which the thought processes are confused, disconnected, or disorganized. Rate only on the basis of integration of the verbal products of the patient; do not rate on the basis of the patient's subjective impression of his own level of functioning.	1	2	3	4	5	6	7	8

5. *Guilt Feelings*—Overconcern or remorse for past behavior. Rate on the basis of the patient's subjective experiences of guilt as evidenced by verbal report with appropriate affect; do not infer guilt feelings from depression, anxiety, or neurotic defenses.	1	2	3	4	5	6	7	8
6. *Tension*—Physical and motor manifestations of tension, nervousness, and heightened activation level. Tension should be rated solely on the basis of physical signs and motor behavior and not on the basis of subjective experiences of tension reported by the patient.	1	2	3	4	5	6	7	8
7. *Mannerisms and Posturing*—Unusual and unnatural motor behavior, the type of motor behavior which causes certain mental patients to stand out in a crowd of normal people. Rate only abnormality of movements; do not rate simple heightened motor activity. Do not rate movements of tardive dyskinesia.	1	2	3	4	5	6	7	8
8. *Grandiosity*—Exaggerated self-opinion, conviction of unusual ability, or powers. Rate only on the basis of patient's statements about self or self-in-relation-to-others, not on the basis of demeanor in the interview situation.	1	2	3	4	5	6	7	8
9. *Depressive Mood*—Despondency in mood, sadness. Rate only degree of despondency; do not rate on the basis of inferences concerning depression based upon general retardation and somatic complaints.	1	2	3	4	5	6	7	8

Continued

Subject ______________________________

Rater ______________________________

Date ______________________________

	Not Present	Very Mild	Mild	Moderate	Moderate-Severe	Severe	Very Severe	Not Assessed
10. *Hostility*—Animosity, contempt, belligerence, disdain for other people outside the interview situation. Rate solely on the basis of the verbal report of feelings and actions of the patient toward others; do not infer hostility from neurotic defenses, anxiety, or somatic complaints. (Rate attitude toward interviewer under "uncooperativeness.")	1	2	3	4	5	6	7	8
11. *Suspiciousness*—Belief (delusional or otherwise) that others have now, or have had in the past, malicious or discriminatory intent toward the patient. On the basis of verbal report, rate only those suspicions which are currently held, whether they concern past or present circumstances.	1	2	3	4	5	6	7	8
12. *Hallucinatory Behavior*—Perceptions without normal external stimulus correspondence. Rate only those experiences which are reported to have occurred within the last week and which are described as distinctly different from the thought and imagery processes of normal people.	1	2	3	4	5	6	7	8

13. *Motor Retardation*—Reduction in energy level evidenced in slowed movements. Rate on the basis of observed behavior of the patient only; do not rate on the basis of patient's subjective impression of own energy level.	1	2	3	4	5	6	7	8
14. *Uncooperativeness*—Evidence of resistance, unfriendliness, resentment, and lack of readiness to cooperate with the interviewer. Rate only on the basis of the patient's attitude and responses to the interviewer and the interview situation; do not rate on the basis of reported resentment or uncooperativeness outside the interview situation.	1	2	3	4	5	6	7	8
15. *Unusual Thought Content*—Unusual, odd, strange, or bizarre thought content. Rate here the degree of unusualness, not the degree of disorganization of thought process.	1	2	3	4	5	6	7	8
16. *Blunted Affect*—Reduced emotional tone, apparent lack of normal feeling or involvement.	1	2	3	4	5	6	7	8
17. *Excitement*—Heightened emotional tone, agitation, increased reactivity.	1	2	3	4	5	6	7	8
18. *Disorientation*—Confusion or lack of proper association for person, place, or time.	1	2	3	4	5	6	7	8

FIGURE 2.2 — GLOBAL ASSESSMENT SCALE	
Rate the patient's lowest level of functioning in the last week by selecting the *lowest range* which describes his/her functioning on a hypothetical continuum of mental health illness. For example, a patient whose "behavior is considerably influenced by delusions" (range 21-30) should be given a rating in that range even though he/she has "major impairment in several areas" (range 31-40). Use intermediary levels when appropriate (eg, 35, 58, 63). Rate actual functioning *independent* of whether or not patient is receiving and may be helped by medication or some other form of treatment.	
________(100–91)	No symptoms, superior functioning in a wide range of activities, life's problems never seem to get out of hand, is sought out by others because of his/her warmth and integrity.
________ (90-81)	Transient symptoms may occur, but good functioning in all areas, interested and involved in a wide range of activities, socially effective, generally satisfied with life, "everyday" worries that only occasionally get out of hand.
________ (80-71)	Minimal symptoms may be present but no more than slight impairment in functioning, varying degrees of "everyday" worries and problems that sometimes get out of hand.
________ (70-61)	Some mild symptoms (eg, depressive mood and mild insomnia) OR some difficulty in several areas of functioning, but generally functioning pretty well, has some meaningful interpersonal relationships and most untrained people would not consider him "sick."

Score	Description
_________ (60-51)	Moderate symptoms OR generally functioning with some difficulty (eg, few friends and flat affect, depressed mood, and pathological self-doubt, euphoric mood and pressure of speech, moderately severe antisocial behavior).
_________ (50-41)	Any serious symptomatology or impairment in functioning that most clinicians would think obviously requires treatment or attention (eg, suicidal preoccupation or gesture, severe obsessional rituals, frequent anxiety attacks, serious antisocial behavior, compulsive drinking).
_________ (40-31)	Major impairment in several areas, such as work, family relations, judgment, thinking, or mood (eg, depressed woman avoids friends, neglects family, unable to do housework) OR some impairment in reality testing or communication (eg, speech is at times obscure, illogical, or irrelevant) OR single serious suicide attempt.
_________ (30-21)	Unable to function in almost all areas (eg, stays in bed all day) OR behavior is considerably influenced by either delusions or hallucinations OR serious impairment in communication (eg, sometimes incoherent or unresponsive) or judgment (eg, acts grossly inappropriately).
_________ (20-11)	Needs some supervision to prevent hurting self and others, or to maintain minimal personal hygiene (eg, repeated suicide attempts, frequently violent, manic excitement, smears feces) OR gross impairment in communication (eg, largely incoherent or mute).
_________ (10-1)	Needs constant supervision for several days to prevent hurting self or others, or makes no attempt to maintain personal hygiene.

- Abnormal Involuntary Movement Scale (AIMS)
- Barnes Akathisia Rating Scale (BARS).

The SAS is a 10-item instrument used to measure drug-induced parkinsonism by assessing rigidity, tremor, and salivation. It is rated on a 5-point scale (0 = complete absence of the condition, 4 = presence of the condition in extreme form). The AIMS is a 12-item instrument that assesses abnormal involuntary movements, specifically tardive dyskinesia, related to antipsychotic therapy. Scoring of the AIMS examination consists of rating the severity of movements in three main areas: facial/oral, extremities, and trunk. This instrument is based on a 5-point scale (0 = none, 4 = severe). The BARS is a 4-item scale used to assess drug-induced akathisia. This scale evaluates objective and subjective features of restlessness and associated distress, which are rated from 0 to 3. There is also a global severity rating on a 6-point scale (0 = absent, 5 = severe). A rating of 2 or more is considered diagnostic for akathisia.

SUGGESTED READING

Kane JM. Pharmacologic treatment of schizophrenia. *Biol Psychiatry*. 1999;46:1396-1408.

Lehman AF. Improving treatment for persons with schizophrenia. *Psychiatr Q*. 1999;70:259-272.

Lehman AF, Steinwachs DM. Patterns of usual care for schizophrenia: initial results for the Schizophrenia Patient Outcomes Research Team (PORT) Client Survey. *Schizophr Bull*. 1998;24:11-20.

Remington G, Chong SA. Conventional versus novel antipsychotics: changing concepts and clinical implications. *J Psychiatry Neurosci*. 1999;24:431-441.

Shen WW. A history of antipsychotic drug development. *Compr Psychiatry*. 1999;40:407-414.

Treatment of schizophrenia 1999. The expert consensus guideline series. *J Clin Psychiatry*. 1999;60(suppl 11):3-80.

3 Second-Generation Antipsychotic Drugs

3

While conventional or traditional antipsychotics exert most of their receptor blockade through dopamine-2 (D_2) receptors, the second-generation antipsychotic drugs (SGADs) may work through different mechanisms. The latter agents have greater affinity for serotonin receptors than for dopamine receptors. The involvement of serotonin in the mechanism of action of SGADs was postulated partly because serotonin is known to exert a regulatory action on dopamine neurons. Studies suggest that serotonin projections inhibit mesolimbic and nigrostriatal dopaminergic activity, and may directly inhibit dopamine release from striatal nerve terminals. The antipsychotic profiles for receptor binding are shown in Figure 3.1.

These medications as a class, however, are heterogeneous in regards to receptor binding and structure activity. The chemical structures for the SGADs are shown in Figure 3.2. The structures of olanzapine and quetiapine are similar to the dibenzodiazepine structure of clozapine. These medications, however, do not possess the superior efficacy of clozapine. Risperidone and ziprasidone are similar in structure, but very different from the other available SGADs.

The SGADs and a summary of dosing information are provided in Table 3.1. Information on the SGADs is listed below in regard to mechanism of action, efficacy, dosing, pharmacokinetics, and adverse effects. Comparative data are presented at the end of the chapter, and information on extrapyramidal symptoms (EPS) and tardive dyskinesia is listed in Chapter 5, *Extrapyramidal Symptoms/Tardive Dyskinesia*.

FIGURE 3.1 — ANTIPSYCHOTIC DRUG PROFILES FOR RECEPTOR-BINDING

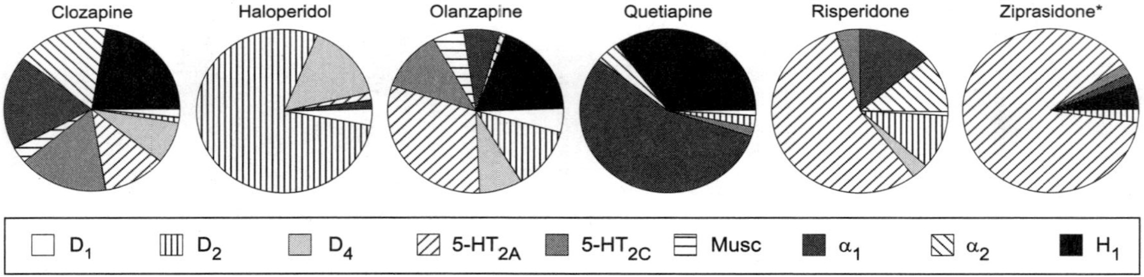

Abbreviations: D, dopamine; 5-HT, serotonin; Musc, muscarinic; H, histamine.

* Investigtional.

Adapted from: Collaborative Working Group on Clinical Evaluations. *J Clin Psychiatry*. 1998;59(suppl 12):7.

FIGURE 3.2 — CHEMICAL STRUCTURES OF SECOND-GENERATION ANTIPSYCHOTIC DRUGS COMPARED WITH HALOPERIDOL

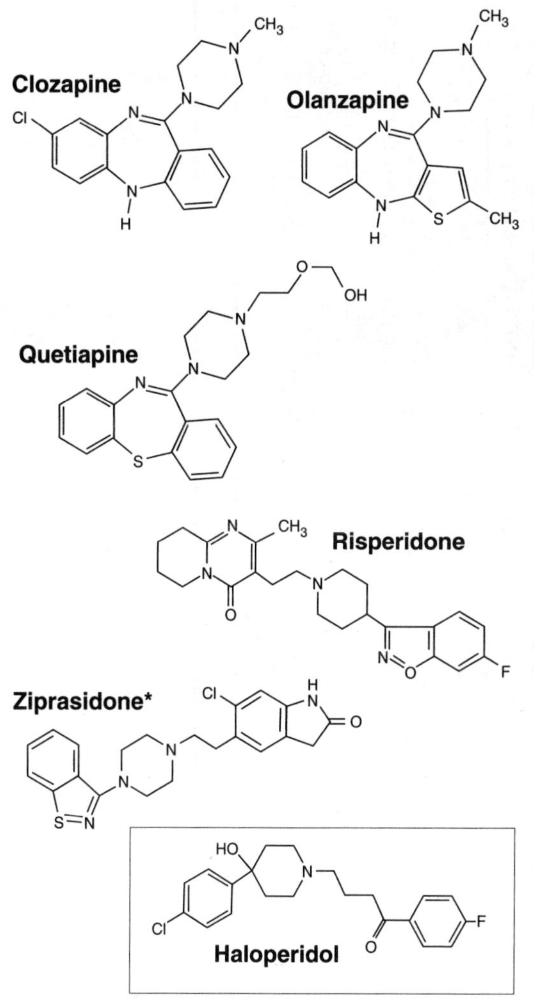

* Investigational.

TABLE 3.1 — SUMMARY OF DOSING INFORMATION FOR SECOND-GENERATION ANTIPSYCHOTIC DRUGS

Antipsychotic Drug	Usual Dosage Range (mg/day)	Available Dosage Forms
Clozapine	300 to 700	25-mg and 100-mg tablets
Risperidone	2 to 6	0.25-mg, 0.5-mg, 1-mg, 2-mg, 3-mg, 4-mg tablets, 1 mg/mL solution
Olanzapine	10 to 20	5-mg, 7.5-mg, 10-mg, 15-mg tablets
Quetiapine	300 to 600	25-mg, 100-mg, 200-mg tablets
Ziprasidone*	40 to 160	—

* Investigational.

Adverse effects in clinical trials occurring with the greatest frequency are listed as well as additional information on other clinically significant or controversial side effects.

Clozapine

3

■ History

Reports of clozapine being effective for psychosis first appeared in the mid 1960s. The use of this agent was controversial because clozapine did not produce EPS, which were thought to be required of an effective antipsychotic at that time. Soon after clozapine began to be widely used in the early 1970s, eight patients in Finland died from agranulocytosis while taking the drug. The use of clozapine declined until the late 1980s, when it reemerged as a treatment for a selected group of treatment-refractory patients. In 1990, after availability was for compassionate use only, clozapine was marketed in the United States. Therapeutic use now includes a weekly laboratory monitoring system.

■ Mechanism of Action

Clozapine is the only agent approved and effective for the treatment of therapy-refractory schizophrenia (see Chapter 8, *Treatment-Resistant Schizophrenia*). A great deal of interest has been generated in understanding what pharmacologic properties of clozapine contribute to its superior efficacy. Clozapine has an increased ratio of D_1 to D_2 antagonism, greater D_3 and D_4 blockade, 5-hydroxytryptamine $(5\text{-HT})_{2A}$ and 5-HT_{2C} antagonistic properties, anticholinergic and antiadrenergic properties, and increased mesolimbic specificity with relative sparing of nigrostriatal dopaminergic neurons.

■ Efficacy

Several trials have consistently found clozapine to be superior to traditional antipsychotics in treatment-refractory patients. Approximately 30% to 50% of patients with treatment-resistant schizophrenia are reported to respond to clozapine treatment. Kane and associates performed the landmark study that helped bring clozapine back into the armamentarium of treatments. His group compared clozapine with chlorpromazine in a stringent study design. Thirty percent of patients responded to clozapine while only 4% of those receiving chlorpromazine responded. Further discussion of treatment resistance can be found in Chapter 8, *Treatment-Resistant Schizophrenia*.

■ Dosing

Due to side effects such as orthostatic hypotension and sedation, titration is recommended for dosing (Table 3.2). Daily dosing should continue on a twice-daily regimen as an effective and tolerable dose level is sought. Most patients will respond to dosing between 300 mg/day and 600 mg/day. In a few instances, patients may respond to doses between 600 mg/day and 900 mg/day; however, this upper range is the maximum recommended dose. Doses higher than 600 mg/day are associated with an increased risk of adverse events, including seizures. Most patients who will benefit from clozapine will typically respond by the end of 8 weeks of therapy.

TABLE 3.2 — DOSING RECOMMENDATIONS FOR CLOZAPINE	
Initiation	12.5 mg qd or bid
Titration	Increase by 25- to 50-mg/day increments
Target	300 to 450 mg/day by the end of 2 weeks

A consensus panel of the National Institute of Mental Health has recommended that if a patient is responding well to treatment with clozapine, withdrawal from the medication should be avoided unless it is medically warranted. Abrupt withdrawal of clozapine may lead to a rebound phenomenon that may be attributed to the cholinergic component of clozapine. Cholinergic rebound after the withdrawal of medication typically is associated with somatic symptoms such as: 3

- Malaise
- Agitation
- Insomnia
- Restlessness
- Anorexia
- Nausea.

The propensity for the rapid onset of these withdrawal symptoms has been linked to the relatively short elimination half-life of clozapine and by the fact that it dissociates from its target receptors more rapidly than other antipsychotics. Aside from somatic symptoms, withdrawal from clozapine also may result in a recurrence of psychotic symptoms. If a patient has not taken clozapine for more than 2 days since the last dose, it is recommended that clozapine be reinitiated with 12.5 mg to 25 mg once or twice daily. If that dose is well tolerated, it may be feasible to titrate patients back to a therapeutic dose more quickly than is recommended for initial treatment. In patients who have previously experienced respiratory or cardiac complications with initial dosing, the dose should be retitrated with extreme caution after even 24 hours of discontinuation.

■ Pharmacokinetics

Clozapine is well absorbed (90% to 95%) and is not affected by the administration of food. It is 97%

plasma protein bound and undergoes extensive first-pass metabolism, resulting in an oral bioavailability of about 50%. The major metabolite of clozapine is *N*-desmethylclozapine (norclozapine), an active metabolite with lower potency than the parent compound but one that may contribute to the bone marrow suppression. Clozapine is metabolized mostly by the cytochrome P450 (CYP450) enzyme 1A2, but 2D6 and 3A4 also play a small role in metabolism of this agent (see Chapter 10, *Drug Interactions With Antipsychotics*). The mean elimination half-life of clozapine after steady-state dosing is 12 hours.

A clozapine dose of 300 mg/day at steady state will typically produce a plasma concentration between 200 ng/mL and 600 ng/mL. Plasma concentrations above 350 ng/mL have been found to be associated with a greater likelihood of response.

■ Adverse Effects

The most frequently occurring side effects from clinical trials are listed in Table 3.3. Information pertaining to treatment recommendations for anticholinergic effects can be found in Chapter 4, *Conventional Antipsychotic Drugs.*

Hematologic Side Effects

Current estimates are that agranulocytosis will develop in approximately 0.8% of patients treated with clozapine. Agranulocytosis is clinically defined as a granulocyte count of less than 500/mm^3, whereas neutropenia is defined as a neutrophil count of less than 1000/mm^3, and leukopenia, as a white blood cell (WBC) count of less than 3500/mm^3. The etiology of agranulocytosis is undetermined; however, it is believed to be immunologically mediated and is not mediated by dosing levels. Risk factors associated with the development of agranulocytosis are:

TABLE 3.3 — ADVERSE EFFECTS OF CLOZAPINE	
Side Effect	**Patients Experiencing Side Effect (%)**
Drowsiness/sedation	39
Salivation	31
Tachycardia	25
Dizziness/vertigo	19
Constipation	14
Hypotension	9
Headache	7
Sweating	6
Dry mouth	6
Syncope	6
Tremor	6
Physicians' Desk Reference. 54th ed. Montvale, NJ: Medical Economics Company, Inc; 2000:2008-2012.	

- Increasing age
- Female gender
- Coadministration with other drugs causing hematologic complications
- Ashkenazi Jewish descent
- African American race.

The period of greatest risk for developing agranulocytosis is within the first 6 months after initiation of therapy. This is the rationale behind the Food and Drug Administration's (FDA) mandate for weekly blood monitoring for the first 6 months. Thereafter, the frequency of monitoring is mandated to be every other week.

The clinical presenting symptoms of early stages of agranulocytosis include:

- Lethargy
- Weakness
- Fever
- Sore throat.

If the WBC count falls to below 3000/mm^3 or the absolute neutrophil count (ANC) to below 1500/mm^3, therapy with clozapine should be interrupted immediately. In a patient with a drop in WBC count to below 2000/mm^3 or an ANC below 1000/mm^3, clozapine should be discontinued and not be reinstated in the future.

Sedation

Drowsiness/sedation, as shown in Table 3.3, is the most frequently occurring side effect of clozapine therapy. It is usually transient and mild in the initial stages of therapy. Sedation is caused primarily by clozapine's antagonism of histamine $(H)_1$ receptors. Precautions to take in order to minimize clozapine-associated sedation include:

- Use of a minimal drug dose
- Bedtime drug administration
- Avoidance of other central nervous system (CNS) depressants.

Hypersalivation

Although salivation is reported in package labeling to occur in about one third of patients treated with clozapine, the reported incidence varies from 0% to 80%. Although the mechanism of hypersalivation is unknown, one explanation is that clozapine may act as an agonist at the muscarinic $(M)_4$ receptor leading to cholinergic activity and excess salivation. Nonetheless, subjective complaints of hypersalivation in clozapine-treated patients may not correlate with measured salivary flow rates. There is little systematic research on treatments for hypersalivation. Its severity often decreases over time during clozapine treatment. A few treatments have been found to be effective, but not in all instances (Table 3.4). These medications should only be used if behavioral programs (ie, initiating chewing gum) are not effective. It is not advisable to treat nocturnal salivation medically. 3

TABLE 3.4 — RECOMMENDED TREATMENTS OF HYPERSALIVATION
• Sugar-free gum • Clonidine • Low-dose benztropine or other anticholinergic • Low-dose benztropine + terazosin combination

Cardiovascular and Respiratory Effects

Tachycardia is a relatively common side effect of clozapine treatment, occurring in about 25% of patients. Tachycardia may be related to rebound effects from related hypotension as well as clozapine-associated anticholinergic properties and its elevation of plasma norepinephrine. Tachycardia is usually transient but may require treatment with a peripheral beta-blocking agent. Rarely, the tachycardia can be related to a type of rapid ventricular tachycardia known as torsade de pointes.

Orthostatic hypotension is often self-limiting and occurs transiently during clozapine initiation and titration. Orthostasis may occur with or without syncope; about 6% of patients will experience fainting. Dihydroergotamine has been used to alleviate orthostatic hypotension; however, there have been rare reports of respiratory arrest and cardiac arrest with the combination. Education about hypotension and advising the patient to rise slowly from a sitting or supine position are important and should be the mainstay of treatment during titration of the drug.

There are a few case reports of clozapine-associated cardiomyopathy and cardiorespiratory arrest. These reports have included patients with and without cardiac histories. Most of these cases involved coadministration of other agents (ie, benzodiazepines), further complicating interpretation of any causal relationship between clozapine and cardiorespiratory complications. Coadministration of benzodiazepines during initiation of clozapine should be avoided, if possible.

Seizures

The risk of seizure is dose-related in patients taking clozapine. The risk of seizure occurrence is 1% to 2% at doses less than 300 mg/day, similar to traditional antipsychotics. The risk of seizure is 3% to 4% at 300 mg/day to 600 mg/day doses and is 5% at doses greater than 600 mg/day. Possible risk factors include:

- Rapid dose titration
- Previous history of neurologic abnormalities or preexisting seizure disorder
- Concomitant use of epileptogenic drugs.

Dosing above 600 mg/day may warrant a baseline electroencephalogram (EEG). Types of seizures that may occur usually include:

- Tonic-clonic
- Complex partial
- Simple partial.

These seizures are usually preceded by myoclonic jerking. Decreasing the clozapine dose or adding an anticonvulsant, such as valproate or phenytoin, is effective treatment for preventing future seizure activity. Patients who are experiencing myoclonus should be monitored closely and possibly treated with an anticonvulsant to avoid a tonic-clonic seizure.

Weight Gain

Weight gain is a side effect associated with most antipsychotics. Clozapine, however, is associated with the greatest amount of weight gain among all of the antipsychotic agents available. An average weight gain after 10 weeks of treatment is about 4.5 kg (9.9 lb). After 12 weeks of treatment, over two thirds of patients on clozapine will gain about 4 kg to 6 kg (8.8 lb to 13.2 lb), and 20% of patients will gain over 10% of their baseline body weight. There has been no direct correlation between dosing and amount of weight gain. Nutrition counseling and exercise are the two most important recommendations that can be made to help reduce the amount of weight gain with this medication.

Urinary Incontinence

Urinary incontinence occurs in about 1% of patients taking clozapine but is thought to be under reported because of the embarrassing nature of the adverse effect. Although the mechanism of urinary incontinence is not known, it is generally believed to occur due to the adrenergic antagonism of clozapine. This may lead to urinary incontinence through a mechanism leading to deceased internal bladder sphincter tone. Ephedrine, an alpha-adrenergic agonist, has been found to be effective in preventing urinary incontinence, as has desmopressin.

Risperidone

■ History and Mechanism of Action

Risperidone, a benzisoxazole derivative, was first marketed in the United States in 1994. It has high binding affinity to both 5-HT_{2A} and D_2 receptors. Additionally, it binds to alpha $(\alpha)_1$ and α_2 receptors, with little blockade of cholinergic receptors.

■ Efficacy

Multicenter clinical trials that led to the FDA approval of risperidone found that it has efficacy that is at least equal to that of haloperidol and produces significantly fewer EPS. The US results of the United States–Canadian collaborative investigation were reported by Marder and Meibach in 1994. They reported that 6 mg/day of risperidone is superior to 20 mg daily of haloperidol. Fifty-seven percent of patients on 6 mg/day of risperidone were found to have a 20% decrease in symptoms as measured by the Positive and Negative Syndrome Scale. In comparison, only 30% receiving haloperidol and 22% receiving placebo also had this symptom reduction. EPS required that 47% of haloperidol-treated patients be treated with antiparkinsonian medication, while only 20% of those on risperidone at 6 mg/daily required treatment.

■ Dosing

The initial package labeling for risperidone recommended that patients were to be treated with 1 mg bid on the first day, 2 mg bid on the second day, and 3 mg bid by the third day of treatment. Since the drug's introduction, it has been found that once-daily dosing is more appropriate. Additionally, new literature emerged since that time reporting that most patients should not be initially titrated to 6 mg/day. Doses between 2 mg/day and 6 mg/day are more efficacious than higher doses. Thus patients should be treated with dosing in this range. Dosing should be initiated between 0.25 mg/day to 1 mg/day and titrated to between 2 mg/day to 4 mg/day in a few days. Some patients may require a slower titration. The safety of risperidone has not been evaluated above 16 mg/day. EPS are dose related; therefore, patients treated with above 6 mg/day will have a greater likelihood of EPS. Patients should receive a trial at least 4 to 6 weeks to maximize likelihood of response.

3

■ Pharmacokinetics

Risperidone is well absorbed and the relative oral bioavailability from a tablet is 94%. Administration with food does not affect the rate or extent of absorption of risperidone. Thus the drug can be given without regard to meals. Risperidone is extensively metabolized in the liver by CYP450 2D6 to a major active metabolite, 9-hydroxyrisperidone. This metabolite is approximately equal with respect to efficacy and receptor binding. Consequently, the clinical effect of the drug probably results from the combined effects of these compounds. The plasma protein binding of risperidone is 90% and the active metabolite is 70%. The half-life of risperidone is approximately 3 hours, while 9-hydroxyrisperidone has an elimination half-life of about 22 hours. This allows for once-daily dosing of risperidone. Plasma concentrations of either active compound have not yielded clinical information on blood levels and their relationships to response.

■ Adverse Effects

Spontaneously reported adverse effects from clinical trials are listed in Table 3.5. Data on EPS can be found in the section entitled *Comparative Data Among Second-Generation Antipsychotic Drugs*, this chapter.

Cardiovascular

Because of risperidone's alpha-blocking activity, orthostatic hypotension may occur. Orthostasis may be associated with dizziness, tachycardia, and in some

TABLE 3.5 — ADVERSE EFFECTS OF RISPERIDONE	
Side Effect	**Patients Experiencing Side Effects (%)**
Insomnia	26
Agitation	22
Headache	14
Anxiety	12
Rhinitis	10
Constipation	7
Nausea	6
Dyspepsia	5
Vomiting	5
Abdominal pain	4

Physicians' Desk Reference. 54th ed. Montvale, NJ: Medical Economics Company, Inc; 2000:1453-1457.

patients, syncope. Syncope occurs rarely, in approximately 0.2% of patients. Tachycardia has been reported to occur in approximately 3% of patients. Orthostatic hypotension is generally seen during the initial dose titration and is usually transient. Risperidone and its metabolite may, in rare cases, lengthen the QT interval. Clinical sequela in known cases is rare; however, risperidone should be used with caution in patients with congenital prolongation in QT, electrolyte imbalance, or concomitant use with other drugs that prolong the QT interval.

Prolactin-Related Adverse Effects

Dopamine receptor antagonists increase prolactin production by inhibiting the action of dopamine on D_2 receptors in the pituitary. Risperidone causes a dose-dependent elevation of plasma prolactin levels of similar magnitude to those observed with haloperidol. Adverse effects related to prolactin elevation, such as amenorrhea, galactorrhea, gynecomastia, and ejaculatory and erectile dysfunction, appear to increase in a dose-related fashion. However, no direct correlation between plasma levels and adverse effects has been identified. At doses lower than 6 mg/day, approximately 8% of women and men will report menstrual or sexual changes. At doses greater than 6 mg/day, more patients may experience prolactin-related problems.

Weight Gain

Risperidone is associated with increased body weight in adults. An average weight gain of 2.8 kg (6.2 lb) occurred after 8 weeks of treatment in adult patients randomized to receive 2 mg, 6 mg, 10 mg, or 16 mg of risperidone in the landmark trials. In a meta-analysis of 78 studies published between 1966 and 1997, risperidone-related weight gain was estimated to be 2.1 kg (4.6 lb) after 10 weeks of treatment. No significant correlation has been found between weight gain and risperidone dose or plasma concentration. Eighteen percent of patients are expected to gain more than 7% of body weight during risperidone therapy. Risperidone treatment is associated with lower weight gain than olanzapine or clozapine treatment.

Olanzapine

■ History and Mechanism of Action

Olanzapine has a pharmacologic profile of activity similar to that of clozapine. In preclinical studies, olanzapine demonstrated a range of receptor affinities distinct from those of conventional antipsychotics and generally comparable to those of clozapine. However, in clinical trials, olanzapine has not been found to be as efficacious for treatment-resistant schizophrenia as is clozapine (see Chapter 8, *Treatment-Resistant Schizophrenia*). Olanzapine has greater affinity for 5-HT_{2A} than for D_2 receptors. In addition, the compound has affinity at the binding sites of D_4, D_3, 5-HT_3, 5-HT_6, H_1, α_1-adrenergic receptors, and $M_{1\text{-}5}$ receptors.

■ Efficacy

Both American and international multicenter studies comparing olanzapine with haloperidol have found that olanzapine is effective in doses of 5.5 mg/day to 20 mg/day. Efficacy with respect to positive symptoms is equivalent to that of haloperidol. Olanzapine's efficacy regarding negative symptoms has been found to be equivalent or superior to that of haloperidol. The clinical trials that brought olanzapine to market compared a low (mean 6.6 mg/day), moderate (11.6 mg/day), and high dose (16.3 mg/day) of olanzapine. There were no significant differences in efficacy among dosage groups. However, the highest dose range appeared to offer the greatest benefit for both positive and negative symptoms compared with haloperidol.

■ Dosing

The recommended dosing for olanzapine is a once-daily dose beginning with 5 mg to 10 mg daily and reaching a target dose of 10 mg/day within several days. Dose increments/decrements are recommended to be 5 mg/day with a maximum dose of 15 mg/day to 20 mg/day. Since its introduction, the recommended dose of 10 mg/day has gravitated upward. The mean dose being utilized currently in the United States is around 18 mg/day. A few case reports have reported the use of olanzapine at doses of up to 40 mg/day. Clinical trials are under way to evaluate the efficacy and safety of higher dosing of olanzapine; however, there are currently no large-scale safety data reporting the use of doses above 20 mg/day. Such doses should be used with caution.

■ Pharmacokinetics

Olanzapine is well absorbed following oral administration and can be given without regard to meals. The plasma protein binding of olanzapine is approximately 93%. Olanzapine is extensively metabolized in the liver to a number of inactive metabolites. The primary processes of metabolism are glucuronidation and demethylation by CYP450 1A2 (see Chapter 10, *Drug Interactions With Antipsychotics*). There is little metabolism of olanzapine occurring by the CYP450 2D6 pathway. The elimination half-life is approximately 31 hours; thus patients can be dosed once daily. Plasma drug levels have not been found to correlate with response, although there has been little work done in that area. The mean plasma concentration in males is approximately 35 ng/mL and 70 ng/mL in females after 8 weeks of treatment at 25-mg/day doses. Differences in plasma concentrations may be due to a slower metabolism or larger volume of distribution in women.

■ Adverse Effects

Table 3.6 lists spontaneously reported adverse effects as seen in clinical trials. Data on EPS can be found at the end of this chapter in the comparative data section.

■ Cardiovascular

Hypotension is reported to occur in 5% to 7% of patients taking olanzapine. Tachycardia occurs in approximately 4% of patients. Syncope was reported to occur in 0.6% of olanzapine-treated patients in

TABLE 3.6 — ADVERSE EFFECTS OF OLANZAPINE	
Side Effect	**Patients Experiencing Side Effect** (%)
Somnolence	26
Agitation	23
Insomnia	20
Headache	17
Nervousness	16
Hostility	15
Dizziness	11
Rhinitis	10
Constipation	9
Dry mouth	7
Physicians' Desk Reference. 54th ed. Montvale, NJ: Medical Economics Company, Inc; 2000:1649-1657.	

phase II and III studies. The risk of orthostatic hypotension usually occurs within the initial dosing period and may be minimized by initiating therapy with a 5-mg daily dose. A more gradual titration to the target dose should be considered if hypotension occurs. Olanzapine should be used with caution in patients with known cardiovascular disease.

■ Transaminase Elevations

In placebo-controlled studies, clinically significant alanine aminotransferase (ALT/SGPT) elevations of greater than or equal to 3 times the upper limit of the normal range were observed in 2% of patients taking olanzapine. Also, during premarketing studies, the incidence of ALT elevations was 2%, but they were not associated with jaundice or other symptoms attributable to liver impairment. Transient increases may be seen but usually normalize with olanzapine continuation. One report of a patient with hepatitis C found persistent enzyme elevations for 4 months following discontinuation of olanzapine.

3

■ Weight Gain

Olanzapine, due to its propensity to block 5-HT_{2c} and H_1 receptors, may cause significant weight gain. In long-term trials (> 1 year), weight gain has ranged from 3.46 kg to 12.06 kg (7.6 lb to 26.6 lb). After 10 weeks of therapy with olanzapine, estimated weight gain is approximately 4.1 kg (9.0 lb). Thirty percent to 40% of patients can be expected to gain over 7% of their body weight during olanzapine treatment. There is some evidence that weight gain with olanzapine may be related to dose, with larger gains occurring at higher doses. A few case reports have found elevated lipids and fasting blood glucose levels occurring during olanzapine treatment. This is usually seen in people who have gained weight, but has been reported in some patients in whom no weight gain has occurred.

Quetiapine

■ History and Mechanism of Action

Structurally, quetiapine is related to clozapine and olanzapine. Quetiapine has high affinity for 5-HT_{2A} receptors and lower affinity for D_1 and D_2 receptors. This agent has some affinity for α_1 and α_2 receptors and H_1 receptors and very little for muscarinic receptors.

■ Efficacy

The efficacy of quetiapine for the treatment of psychosis was established in three short-term controlled trials. One trial evaluated five fixed doses (75 mg/day, 150 mg/day, 300 mg/day, 600 mg/day, and 750 mg/day) vs placebo. The maximum efficacy was found to occur at 300 mg/day. Another fixed-dose trial evaluated 50 mg/day vs 450 mg/day and found the higher dose to be superior. Additionally, quetiapine was tested in a flexible-dose study (< 250 mg/day vs 250 mg/day to 750 mg/day). The mean dose was 360 mg/day in the high-dose group and 209 mg/day in the low-dose group. The greatest efficacy for positive symptoms occurred at doses greater than 250 mg/day. In contrast to the other SGADs, quetiapine has not been shown to be superior to haloperidol in any symptom dimension, such as positive or negative symptoms.

■ Dosing

The dosing recommendations for quetiapine are initiation at a 25-mg dose twice daily with increases by increments of 25 mg to 50 mg bid or tid on the second and third days, as tolerated, to a target dose range of 300 mg/day to 400 mg/day by the fourth day, given two or three times daily. Additional dosage adjustments of 25 mg to 50 mg bid should generally occur at intervals of not less that 2 days. The dose range for efficacy was found in trials to be 150 mg/day to 750 mg/day. The safety and efficacy of quetiapine have not been evaluated above 800 mg/day. The most effective dose appears to be greater than or equal to 300 mg/day.

■ Pharmacokinetics

Quetiapine is rapidly absorbed after oral administration. The bioavailability is marginally increased by administration with food. This agent is 83% bound to plasma proteins and is extensively metabolized by the liver. The enzyme involved with metabolism is the CYP450 3A4 and the two major metabolites are pharmacologically inactive. The elimination half-life is approximately 6 hours; thus quetiapine should be administered 2 to 4 times daily. To date, there are no good data on plasma concentrations and clinical response.

■ Adverse Effects

3

The spontaneously reported adverse effects from landmark clinical trials are listed in Table 3.7. Data on EPS can be found at the end of this chapter under comparative adverse effects.

TABLE 3.7 — ADVERSE EFFECTS OF QUETIAPINE

Side Effect	Patients Experiencing Side Effect (%)
Headache	19
Somnolence	18
Dizziness	10
Constipation	9
Dry mouth	7
Postural hypotension	7
Tachycardia	7
Dyspepsia	6

Physicians' Desk Reference. 54th ed. Montvale, NJ: Medical Economics Company, Inc; 2000:562-566.

Hypothyroidism

In clinical trials, a dose-related decrease in total and free thyroxine (T_4) of approximately 20% was seen in a few patients in the first 2 to 4 weeks of treatment and maintained during chronic therapy. Generally, these changes were of no clinical significance and thyroid-stimulating hormone (TSH) was unchanged in most patients. Others have reported that less than 5% of patients experienced any changes. Approximately 0.4% (10/2386) of patients did experience TSH increases. Six of these patients with TSH increases needed thyroid-replacement therapy.

Cardiovascular

Quetiapine may cause orthostatic hypotension associated with dizziness, tachycardia, and in some patients, syncope. Syncope may occur in approximately 1% of patients treated, usually during the initial dose titration period. The risk of syncope and hypotension may be minimized by limiting the initial dosage to 25 mg bid. QT-wave prolongations and T-wave abnormalities have rarely been reported with quetiapine use.

Cataracts

Within manufacturer labeling, the warning for cataract development appears in bold ink, as required by the FDA. The warning states that the development of cataracts was observed in chronic dog studies and that examinations of the lens by slit-lamp examination or other appropriately sensitive method to detect cataract formation is recommended at initiation and at 6-month intervals thereafter. There have been lens changes occurring in humans after long-term therapy, but a causal relationship has not been established. To date, there are no human reports of cataract formation during quetiapine therapy. The standard of care in the field in regard to this potential adverse effect is to ensure there is an ophthalmoscopic examination performed within the previous 6 months prior to initiation, with follow-up examinations, if deemed necessary.

Transaminase Elevations

Asymptomatic transient and reversible elevations in plasma transaminases (primarily ALT) have been reported. Six percent of patients treated with quetiapine in clinical trials were found to have elevations of greater than 3 times the upper limits of the normal reference range. Hepatic enzyme elevations generally occurred within the first 3 weeks of drug treatment and returned to pretreatment levels after discontinuation of quetiapine.

Weight Gain

Quetiapine appears to be associated with less weight gain than clozapine or olanzapine. To date, there are insufficient data available to make meaningful comparisons with other antipsychotics.

Ziprasidone

■ History and Mechanism of Action

Ziprasidone was developed within a structure-activity investigation intended to find a compound that potently blocks D_2 receptors but binds with even greater affinity to central 5-HT_{2A} receptors. As a result, ziprasidone has a binding affinity ratio of 11:1 for 5-HT_{2A} and D_2. Ziprasidone also binds with relatively high affinity for 5-HT_{2C}, 5-HT_{1D}, α_1-adrenergic receptors, and D_1 receptors.

■ Efficacy

Ziprasidone is currently under consideration for FDA approval. Several short-term clinical trials have been completed using this drug. In double-blind, fixed-dose, placebo-controlled studies, ziprasidone was significantly more effective than placebo in improving overall psychopathology in patients with schizophrenia and schizoaffective disorder.

■ Dosing

Although manufacturer guidelines are not yet available, ziprasidone appears to be most effective in the dose range of 80 mg/day to 160 mg/day.

■ Pharmacokinetics

Ziprasidone is rapidly absorbed after oral administration, and absorption is increased by 100% with food. Ziprasidone is highly bound (> 99%) to plasma proteins. It is extensively metabolized in the liver with no active metabolites. Although the specific isoenzyme metabolism is not fully elucidated, this agent does not appear to inhibit any of the enzyme pathways and may be metabolized by CYP450 3A3/4. No data are available to date regarding plasma levels and response.

■ Adverse Effects

The adverse effects listed in Table 3.8 were spontaneously reported from a pivotal clinical trial. There have been a few cases of QT prolongation with ziprasidone use which are currently under investigation.

Comparative Data Among Second-Generation Antipsychotic Drugs

■ Efficacy

Few data exist in regard to efficacy by direct head-to-head comparison studies between the SGADs. Leucht and others completed a useful meta-analysis of currently published trials comparing the SGADs, other than clozapine, to placebo or haloperidol. They found all of the drugs to be more efficacious than placebo. Risperidone and olanzapine were more effective than haloperidol for global psychopathology and negative symptoms. All medications were better with regard to EPS. Other data suggests that risperidone

TABLE 3.8 — ADVERSE EFFECTS OF ZIPRASIDONE*	
Side Effect	**Patients Experiencing Side Effect (%)**
Headache	22
Somnolence	14
Insomnia	11
Nausea	10
Constipation	9
Dizziness	8
Dyspepsia	8
Diarrhea	5
Asthenia	5
* Investigational.	
Daniel DG, et al. *Neuropharmacology*. 1999;20:491-505.	

3

may be more effective for positive symptoms compared to haloperidol, but this has not been found for the other SGADs, excluding clozapine (Table 3.9).

Risperidone, olanzapine, and quetiapine are similar in efficacy in overall symptomatology. There appear to be some differences in efficacy in subfactors of the Brief Psychiatric Rating Scale (such as positive, negative, and depressive symptoms) between these drugs. Large-scale, investigator-initiated, comparative trials are needed to clarify these variances. There are important differences, however, between these medications in terms of pharmacokinetics, cost, and adverse effects.

TABLE 3.9 — EFFICACY OF SECOND-GENERATION ANTIPSYCHOTIC DRUGS COMPARED WITH HALOPERIDOL			
Drug	Global Symptoms	Positive Symptoms	Negative Symptoms
Risperidone	+	+	+
Olanzapine	+	=	+
Quetiapine	=	=	= / –
Ziprasidone*	=	=	=
Key: + (superior), = (no difference), – (not as good).			
* Investigational.			

■ Adverse Effects

Extrapyramidal

It is well accepted that *in vitro* binding affinity of antipsychotics to the D_2 receptors predicts the likelihood of causing EPS. This relationship has been supported by *in vivo* radioligand binding studies with positron emission tomography. Blockade of 5-HT_{2A} receptors may mitigate against the EPS of these drugs. The comparative D_2 receptor blockades are shown in Figure 3.3

Much of the clinical advantage favoring SGADs comes from the fact that there is a wider separation between doses that cause EPS compared with effective doses of these drugs compared with conventional antipsychotics (Figure 3.4). This property may lead to a better quality of life and greater compliance in people who are prescribed these medications.

Clinically, the rates of EPS are comparable to the *in vitro* binding. Clozapine is associated with little to no EPS, and quetiapine has been found to have no greater rates of EPS than placebo. Olanzapine and risperidone both cause EPS less often than do con-

FIGURE 3.3 — DOPAMINE-2 RECEPTOR BLOCKADE OF ANTIPSYCHOTICS*

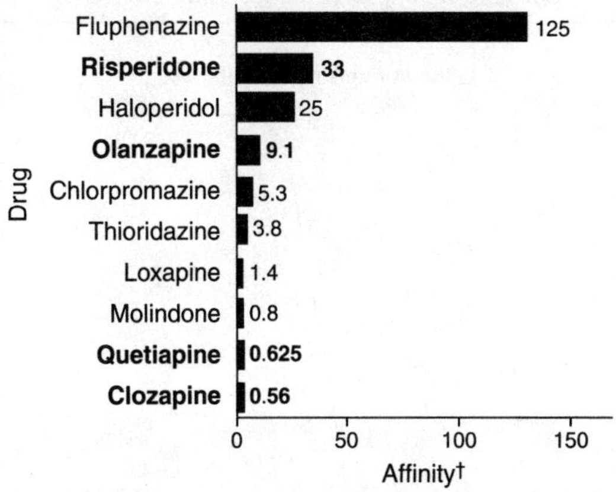

* Affinity data were compiled from: Richelson E, Nelson A. *Eur J Pharmacol.* 1984;103:197-204; Moore NA, et al. *Curr Opin Invest Drugs.* 1993;2:281-293; Hyttel J, et al. *Clin Neuropharmacol.* 1992;15:267a-268a.

† $10^{-7} \times 1/K_d$ where K_d = equilibrium dissociation in molarity.

Richelson E. *J Clin Psychiatry*. 1996:57(suppl 11):4-11.

ventional antipsychotics but in a dose-related fashion. Risperidone treatment is associated with parkinsonism rates similar to placebo in doses under 6 mg/day. Doses higher than 6 mg/day are associated with EPS rates of 20% or greater. Parkinsonism with olanzapine is similar to placebo with doses up to 10 mg/day. At higher doses, the rate increases to 20%. Akathisia with olanzapine is significantly higher than with placebo at doses greater than 10 mg/day. Tardive dyskinesia with all the SGADs appears to occur at an incidence of less than 2%, but few long-term follow-up studies are yet available.

FIGURE 3.4 — EXTRAPYRAMIDAL SYMPTOM CURVES FOR CONVENTIONAL AND SECOND-GENERATION ANTIPSYCHOTIC DRUGS

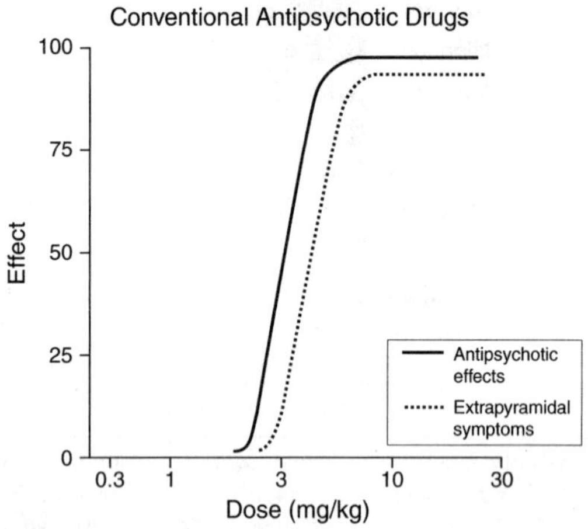

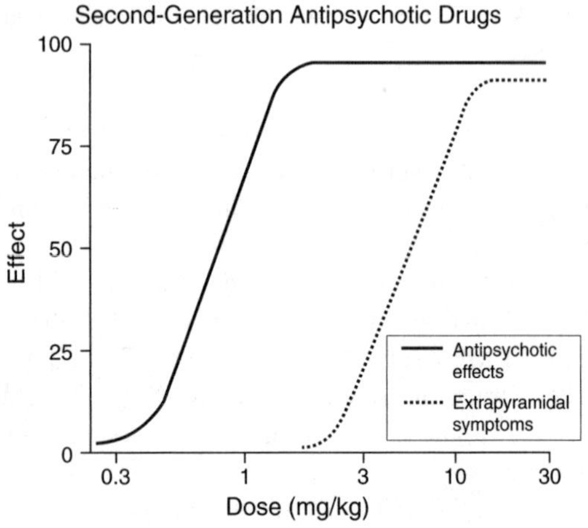

Casey DE. *Int Clin Psychopharmacol*. 1995;10(suppl 3):105-114.

■ Weight Gain

Treatment with conventional antipsychotics has long been noted to cause weight gain. This is also true with the SGADs, which cause comparable, if not greater, weight gain. Weight gain is a serious side effect with potential consequences, including diminished self-image, decreased social interactions, and noncompliance with medication. Health problems associated with obesity include hypertension, diabetes, dyslipidemia, and orthopedic complications, among others. The etiology of weight gain is not completely clear, although it may be mediated by 5-HT_{2C} antagonism and possibly H_1 blockade. Clozapine is associated with the greatest amount of weight gain with olanzapine not far behind. Risperidone and quetiapine also cause weight gain but to a degree more comparable with that caused by high-potency neuroleptics (Figure 3.5).

3

■ Prolactin-Related Adverse Effects/Sexual Dysfunction

Antipsychotics increase prolactin production by inhibiting the action of D_2 receptors in pituitary lactotrophs. This effect occurs within the tuberoinfundibular pathway of the dopamine system. Haloperidol and other conventional antipsychotics increase dopamine concentrations in a dose-dependent fashion. Clozapine and quetiapine do not elevate prolactin levels, while both risperidone and olanzapine do. Problems associated with elevated prolactin levels include:

- Amenorrhea and galactorrhea in women
- Erectile dysfunction, ejaculatory dysfunction, and gynecomastia in men.

Prolactin concentrations with risperidone remain elevated throughout therapy. Prolactin concentrations with olanzapine therapy will usually decrease after several weeks of treatment. Although prolactin lev-

FIGURE 3.5 — WEIGHT GAIN WITH ANTIPSYCHOTIC DRUGS*

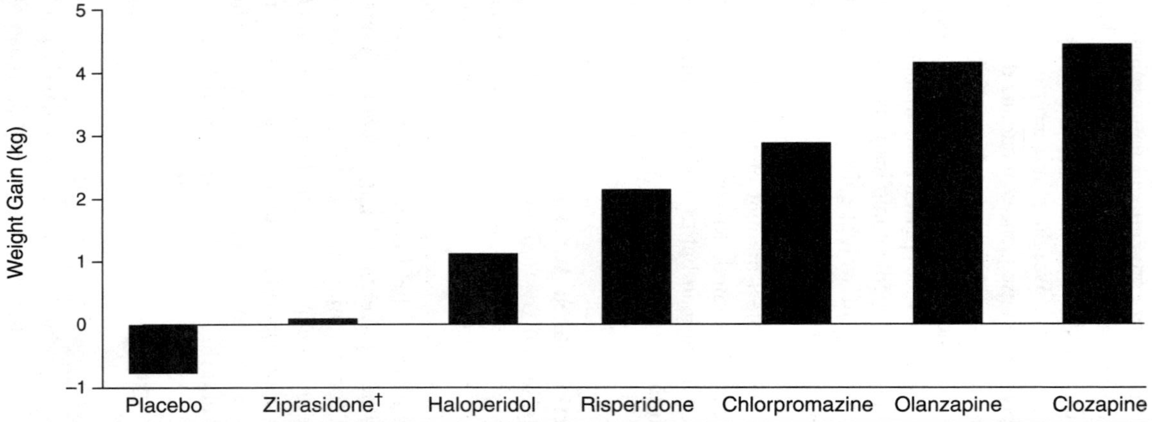

1 kilogram is equivalent to 2.2 pounds.

* Meta-analysis at 10 weeks.

† Investigational.

Adapted from: Allison DB, et al. *Am J Psychiatry*. 1999;156:1690.

els are elevated, these levels have not been found to consistently correlate with adverse effects. The risk for prolactin-related adverse effects in clinical trials is approximately 3% with risperidone and 1% with olanzapine. However, in real-world use, rates of prolactin-related adverse effects may be greater than those seen in short-term clinical trials.

3

■ Other Side Effects

The incidence of other side effects differs among the atypical antipsychotics and to a great extent is predictable from the differences in their respective pharmacologic profiles (Table 3.10).

SUGGESTED READING

Allison DB, Mentore JL, Heo M, et al. Antipsychotic-induced weight gain: a comprehensive research synthesis. *Am J Psychiatry*. 1999;156:1686-1696.

Andersson C, Chakos M, Mailman R, Lieberman J. Emerging roles for novel antipsychotic medications in the treatment of schizophrenia. *Psychiatr Clin North Am*. 1998;21:151-179.

Brown CS, Markowitz JS, Moore TR, Parker NG. Atypical antipsychotics: Part II: Adverse effects, drug interactions, and costs. *Ann Pharmacother*. 1999;33:210-217.

Casey DE. Motor and mental aspects of extrapyramidal syndromes. *Int Clin Psychopharmacol*. 1995;10(suppl 3):105-114.

Collaborative Working Group on Clinical Trial Evaluations. Measuring outcome in schizophrenia: differences among the atypical antipsychotics. *J Clin Psychiatry*. 1998;59(suppl 12):3-9.

Daniel DG, Zimbroff DL, Potkin SG, Reeves KR, Harrigan EP, Lakshminarayanan M. Ziprasidone 80 mg/day and 160 mg/day in the acute exacerbation of schizophrenia and schizoaffective disorders: a 6-week placebo-controlled trial. Ziprasidone Study Group. *Neuropharmacology*. 1999;20:491-505.

TABLE 3.10 — ADVERSE EFFECTS OF SECOND-GENERATION ANTIPSYCHOTIC DRUGS

Drug	Sedation	Anticholinergic Effects	Orthostatic Hypotension
Chlorpromazine	+++	+++	+++
Clozapine	+++	+++	+++
Haloperidol	+	0/+	0/+
Olanzapine	++	++	++
Quetiapine	++	0	+
Risperidone	+	+	+

Key: 0 (absent), + (minimal), ++ (mild), +++ (moderate).

Goff DC, Posever T, Herz L, et al. An exploratory haloperidol-controlled dose-finding study of ziprasidone in hospitalized patients with schizophrenia or schizoaffective disorder. *J Clin Psychopharmacol.* 1998;18:296-304.

Hyttel J, Arnt J, Costall B, et al. Pharmacological profile of the atypical neuroleptic sertindole. *Clin Neuropharmacol.* 1992;15: 267a-268a.

Leucht A, Pitschel-Walz G, Abraham D, Kissling W. Efficacy and extrapyramidal side-effects of the new antipsychotics olanzapine, quetiapine, risperidone, and sertindole compared to conventional antipsychotics and placebo. A meta-analysis of randomized controlled trials. *Schizophr Res.* 1999;35:51-68.

Marder SR, Meibach RC. Risperidone in the treatment of schizophrenia. *Am J Psychiatry.* 1994;151:825-835.

Moore NA, Calligaro DO, Wong DT, et al. The pharmacology of olanzapine and other new antipsychotic agents. Curr Opin Invest Drugs. 1993;2:281-293.

Physicians' Desk Reference. 54th ed. Montvale, NJ: Medical Economics Company, Inc; 2000:562-566, 1453-1457, 1649-1657, 2008-2012.

Purdon SE. Cognitive improvement in schizophrenia with novel antipsychotic medications. *Schizophr Res.* 1999;35(suppl):S51-S60.

Remington G, Kapur S. D2 and 5-HT2 receptor effects of antipsychotics: bridging basic and clinical findings using PET. *J Clin Psychiatry.* 1999;60(suppl 10):15-19.

Richelson E. Preclinical pharmacology of neuroleptics: focus on new generation compounds. *J Clin Psychiatry.* 1996;57(suppl 11):4-11.

Richelson E, Nelson A. Antagonism by neuroleptics of neurotransmitter receptors of normal human brain *in vitro*. *Eur J Pharmacol.* 1984;103:197-204.

Wetterling T, Mussigbrodt HE. Weight gain: side effect of atypical neuroleptics? *J Clin Psychopharmacol.* 1999;19:316-321.

4 Conventional Antipsychotic Drugs

History

Antipsychotic drugs have been in clinical use since the 1950s when chlorpromazine was synthesized in France. It was first used as a preanesthetic agent. Within 2 years of use, it was found to be effective in the treatment of psychotic patients. Many other similar medications followed in the next decade. These medications were commonly referred to as neuroleptics, which meant "causing a neurologic disorder." This name came about due to the profound extrapyramidal symptoms (EPS) they produced. Many believed the induction of motor side effects was necessary, however, for efficacy of the medications.

Mechanism of Action and Structures

All of the conventional antipsychotic agents available are high-affinity dopamine $(D)_2$ receptor antagonists. Among the conventional compounds, although there are some differences in their affinities for D_1 and D_2 receptors, these differences do not appear to be clinically significant. These agents block 65% to 80% of D_2 receptors in the striatum during chronic treatment and block dopamine in the other three dopamine tracts as well.

Phenothiazines, the first chemical class of antipsychotic drugs developed, are tricyclic molecules. Three subtypes of phenothiazines are available:

- Aliphatics
- Piperidines
- Piperazines.

These subtypes differ chemically, depending on the substituent on a ring-nitrogen. The phenothiazines with aliphatic side chains tend to be low-potency compounds (ie, higher equivalent doses are needed to achieve therapeutic effectiveness). Piperidine substitutions have anticholinergic properties and a lower incidence of EPS. Piperazine agents are the most potent of the phenothiazines. Other than the phenothiazines, classes available are:

- Thioxanthenes
- Butyrophenones
- Diphenylbutylpiperidines
- Dihydroindolones
- Dibenzodiazepines (Figure 4.1).

Efficacy and Dosing

All conventional antipsychotics are equivalent in efficacy when used in equipotent doses (see Chapter 2, *Treatment of Schizophrenia*). Interindividual variation does occur between traditional antipsychotics such that a relatively responsive patient may not respond equally to each antipsychotic. Selection of medication should be based on the need to avoid certain side effects based on patient variables or concurrent medical or psychiatric disorders. There are no differences in efficacy between the low- and high-potency agents. Previous family history of response is also helpful in the selection of an agent. Traditional dosage equivalents (expressed in chlorpromazine [CPZ]-equivalent dosages) are the equipotent dosages of any of the traditional antipsychotics compared with 100 mg of CPZ. The usual recommendation for initiation of therapy is 400 CPZ to 600 CPZ equivalents unless the patient's history indicates that this dose may result in unacceptable adverse effects. Maintenance therapy should provide a dose of 300 CPZ to 600 CPZ equivalents for maximum efficacy. In the 1970s and

1980s, large doses were utilized with the belief that larger daily doses were necessary in more severely symptomatic patients. Randomized controlled trials have found no difference in efficacy between recommended and high-dose therapies. Information on available dosage forms and dosing is provided in Table 4.1 and Table 4.2.

Pharmacokinetics

Conventional antipsychotics are generally well absorbed through the gastrointestinal tract and undergo extensive first-pass hepatic metabolism. Food and antacids may decrease absorption. Liquid preparations are absorbed more rapidly and reliably than tablets and capsules. Antipsychotic drugs are generally highly protein bound (85% to 90%). These agents are highly lipophilic; thus they readily cross the blood-brain barrier and attain high concentrations in the brain. Given their high degree of protein and tissue binding, these drugs are not removed efficiently by dialysis. The elimination half-life of most of the conventional antipsychotics is 18 to 40 hours, therefore, most agents can be administered once daily, side effects permitting.

Most of the agents are metabolized in the liver to demethylated and hydroxylated forms. Several of the hydroxyl and desmethyl metabolites of the phenothiazines are active as dopamine antagonists. Chlorpromazine has an active metabolite, 7-hydroxychlorpromazine fluphenazine is metabolized to 7-hydroxyfluphenazine; and thioridazine is metabolized to mesoridazine. Haloperidol, perphenazine, and thioridazine are metabolized by the cytochrome P450 (CYP450) 2D6 isoenzyme (see Chapter 10, *Drug Interactions With Antipsychotics*). The measurement of plasma levels has not correlated well with response. Currently, haloperidol is the only agent on which some

FIGURE 4.1 — STRUCTURE OF CONVENTIONAL ANTIPSYCHOTICS

Aliphatic Phenothiazine

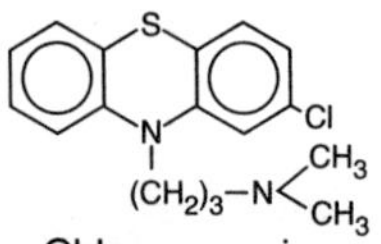

Chlorpromazine

Piperazine Phenothiazines

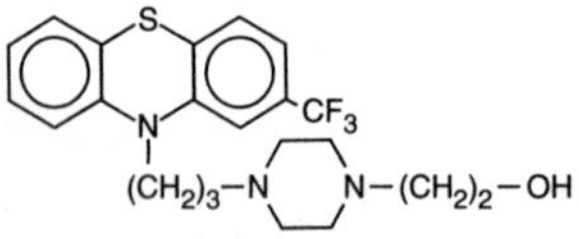

Fluphenazine

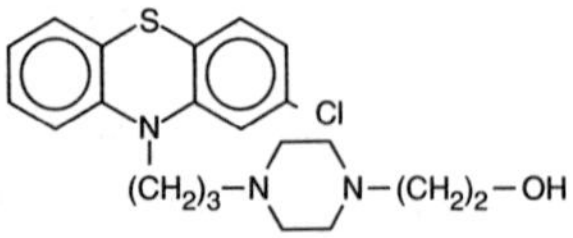

Perphenazine

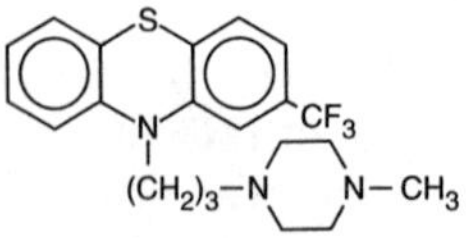

Trifluoperazine

Piperidine Phenothiazines

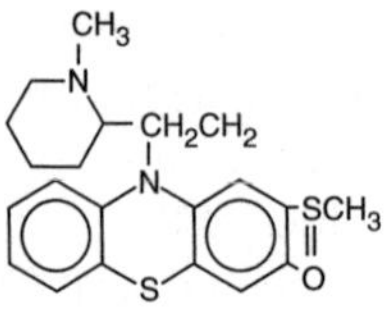

Mesoridazine

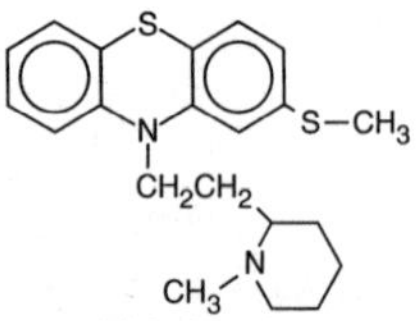

Thioridazine

Thioxanthene

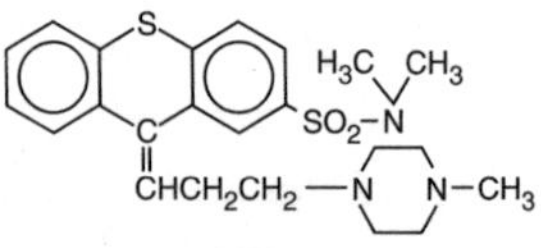

Thiothixene

Butyrophenone

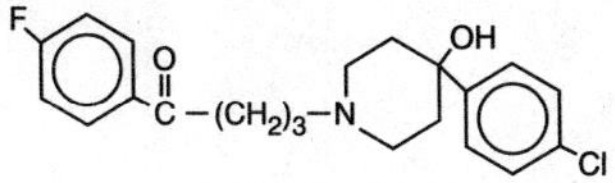

Haloperidol

Dibenzoxazepine

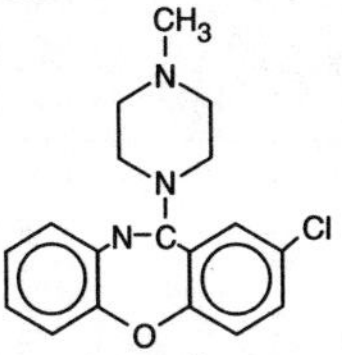

Loxapine

Dihydroindolone

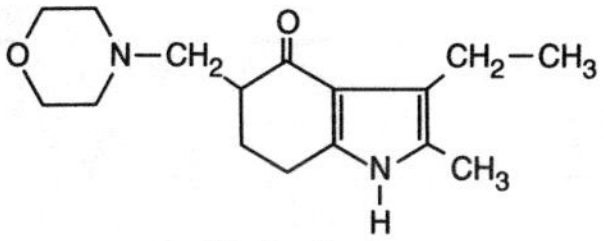

Molindone

Diphenylbutylpiperidine

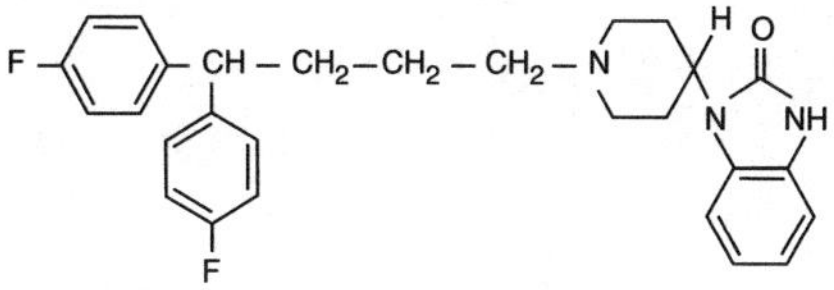

Pimozide

TABLE 4.1 — AVAILABLE PREPARATIONS OF CONVENTIONAL ANTIPSYCHOTIC DRUGS

Drug	**Tablets** (mg)	**Liquid** (mg/mL)	**Parenteral** (mg/mL)	**Other**
Chlorpromazine	10, 25, 50, 100, 200	10/5, 30, 100	25	30-, 75-, 150-mg sustained-release capsules; 25-, 100-mg rectal suppositories
Fluphenazine	1, 2.5, 5, 10	2.5/5, 5	2.5	25 mg/mL decanoate; 25 mg/mL enanthate
Haloperidol	0.5, 1, 2, 5, 10, 20	2	5	50 mg/mL, 100 mg/mL decanoate (intramuscular only)
Loxapine	—	25	50 (intramuscular only)	5-, 10-, 25-, 50-mg capsules
Mesoridazine	10, 25, 50, 100	25	25	—
Molindone	5, 10, 25, 50, 100	20	—	—
Perphenazine	2, 4, 8, 16	16/5	5	—

Pimozide	1, 2	—	—	—
Trifluoperazine	1, 2, 5, 10	10	2	—
Thioridazine	10, 15, 25, 50, 100, 150, 200	25/5, 100/5, 30, 100	—	—
Thiothixene	—	5	—	1-, 2-, 5-, 10-, 20-mg capsules

TABLE 4.2 — DOSING INFORMATION FOR CONVENTIONAL ANTIPSYCHOTIC DRUGS	
Drug	**Dosage Range** (mg/day)
Chlorpromazine	300 to 800
Fluphenazine	2 to 40
Haloperidol	5 to 30
Loxapine	25 to 100
Mesoridazine	150 to 500
Molindone	25 to 100
Perphenazine	8 to 64
Pimozide	1 to 10
Thioridazine	300 to 700
Thiothixene	5 to 40
Trifluoperazine	15 to 30

consistent data on plasma level to response are available. There is evidence that haloperidol levels greater than 5 ng/mL to 10 ng/mL may correspond with clinical antipsychotic effects.

Decanoates

Depot preparations of two antipsychotics (fluphenazine decanoate, fluphenazine enanthate, and haloperidol decanoate) are available in the United States. These are esterified antipsychotics formulated in sesame seed oil for deep intramuscular injection. Because these are long-acting preparations, patients should be exposed to the oral form of the drug prior to their first injection to minimize the possibility of long-acting side effects. With initial dosing, oral supplementation may temporarily be necessary. Care must be taken not to increase the depot preparation too rapidly because steady state is only reached after 4 to 5 dosing intervals.

The pharmacokinetics of the depot agents are useful parameters for strategic dosing. Patients may be dosed with fluphenazine decanoate on a 1-week to 3-week basis, while haloperidol decanoate is usually administered once a month. There is much variability in dosing; however, conversion from oral to depot and maintenance dosing recommendations are listed in Table 4.3.

Based on the above recommendations, a reasonable estimate is that 0.5 mL of fluphenazine decanoate given every 2 weeks is equivalent to 10 mg/day of fluphenazine orally. A maintenance haloperidol decanoate dose of 150 mg every 4 weeks is equivalent to 10 mg/day of oral haloperidol.

Adverse Effects of Conventional Antipsychotic Drugs

Conventional antipsychotics cause a wide range of adverse events, affecting many organ systems. In general, the adverse effects of the low-potency agents are more non-neurologic in nature and the higher potency agents cause most adverse neurologic effects. Most, but not all, of the adverse effects seen with these agents can be categorized by the neurotransmitter system affected (Table 4.4).

Sedation, anticholinergic effects, and cardiovascular effects are all dependent upon the potency of the antipsychotic. The lower-potency agents cause these adverse effects at a higher rate (Table 4.5).

■ Sedation

Sedation is primarily a result of the blockade of histamine $(H)_1$ receptors. The low-potency agents are the most sedating of the conventional antipsychotics.

TABLE 4.3 — DOSING RECOMMENDATIONS FOR DECANOATES		
Drug	**Starting Dose**	**Maintenance Dose**
Haloperidol decanoate	20 × oral haloperidol 100-450 mg/28 days	10-15 × oral haloperidol 50-300 mg/28 days
Fluphenazine decanoate	1.2 × oral fluphenazine 12.5-75 mg/ 7 to 21 days	Based on starting dose and clinical response
Fluphenazine enanthate	12.5-100 mg/7 to 21 days	Based on starting dose and clinical response

TABLE 4.4 — ADVERSE EFFECTS ASSOCIATED WITH RECEPTOR ANTAGONISM	
Receptor	**Adverse Effect**
Histamine-1	Sedation, weight gain
Muscarinic	Urinary retention, dry mouth, blurred vision, constipation, sinus tachycardia, cognition and memory deficits
Alpha-1	Orthostatic hypotension, reflex tachycardia, miosis
Serotonin-2C	Weight gain
Dopamine-2	Extrapyramidal symptoms, hyperprolactinemia/sexual dysfunction

Oversedation may decrease cognitive, perceptual, and motor dysfunction. Thus patients should be warned about driving or operating machinery when first treated with these agents. The entire dose may be given at bedtime to decrease daytime drowsiness. Tolerance to sedation usually develops after several weeks.

TABLE 4.5 — ADVERSE EFFECTS OF CONVENTIONAL ANTIPSYCHOTIC DRUGS

Drug	Sedation	Anticholinergic Effect	Cardiovascular Effect
Chlorpromazine	++++	+++	++++
Fluphenazine	++	++	++
Haloperidol	+	+	+
Loxapine	+++	++	+++
Mesoridazine	+++	+++	+++
Molindone	+	++	++
Perphenazine	++	++	++
Thioridazine	++++	++++	++++
Thiothixene	++	++	++
Trifluoperazine	++	++	++

Key: + (very low), ++ (low), +++ (moderate), ++++ (high).

4

■ Cardiovascular Side Effects

The low-potency agents are more cardiotoxic than the high-potency drugs. Chlorpromazine and thioridazine, in particular, cause prolongation of the QT and PR intervals, blunting of T-waves, and depression of the ST segment. Thus, the piperidine phenothiazines are the most lethal among the antipsychotics in overdose situations. Torsade de pointes has been reported with thioridazine, possibly due to its sulfoxide metabolite, which may cause sudden death. Nonetheless, most electrocardiogram (EKG) changes are not usually clinically significant that occur when normal therapeutic doses are given to physically healthy patients. In patients over 40 years of age, a pretreatment EKG is recommended.

Orthostatic (postural) hypotension, defined as a drop in systolic pressure greater than 20 mm Hg, most frequently occurs with chlorpromazine and thioridazine. Reflex vasoconstriction when rising to a sitting or standing position is inhibited when alpha-adrenergic receptors are blocked. This appears to be caused by a combination of local vasodilatory effects and central inhibition of the vasomotor center, as well as sympatholysis leading to unopposed beta-adrenergic effects. This side effect most frequently occurs when high doses are given via the intramuscular route and during the first few days of oral treatment. Patients usually gain a tolerance to orthostasis within a few days. The primary danger of orthostasis is that patients may fall or faint and injure themselves. Elderly, diabetic patients, and those with preexisting cardiovascular disease may be most predisposed.

When beginning treatment with low-potency agents, the patient should be warned of the adverse effects and advised to rise from bed gradually, sit at first with their legs dangling, wait a minute, and sit or lie down if they feel faint. Additionally, the clinician should measure the patient's blood pressure (supine and standing, separated by several minutes) before and after the first several days of treatment. If hypotension continues to occur, the symptoms can usually be managed by having patients lie down with their feet higher than their head. Support hose may be of benefit. If orthostasis persists, switching to a higher-potency agent or a second-generation antipsychotic drug (SGAD) is warranted. Rarely would volume expansion or vasopressor agents (eg, norepinephrine) be used.

4

■ Anticholinergic Effects

Chlorpromazine, thioridazine, mesoridazine, and trifluoperazine are the most potent anticholinergic agents among the conventional antipsychotics. Anticholinergic effects can be particularly severe if used in the elderly or if low-potency agents are used in combination with other medications possessing this property, such as tricyclic antidepressants or antiparkinsonian agents.

Patients who are troubled by dry mouth should be advised to rinse their mouth out frequently with water and to chew sugar-free gum and candy since with these there is a lower chance of fungal infections and dental caries. Oral lubricants (Xerolube) and ice chips are other treatments. If patients are experiencing constipation, the first treatment should be increases in fluid and dietary fiber intake and exercise, if possible. If not, constipation should be treated with routine laxative preparations, such as Metamucil or docusate sodium. Untreated constipation can lead to paralytic ileus, which may necessitate consultation or referral to outside specialists. Urinary retention may be treated with bethanechol (Urecholine), 20 mg/day to 40 mg/day. However, persistent anticholinergic effects probably warrant a decrease in antipsychotic dose or switching to another agent.

Marked anticholinergic effects may include:

- Cognitive decline
- Severe agitation
- Disorientation
- Hallucinations
- Seizures
- High fever
- Mydriasis.

If these signs or symptoms arise, the causative agent should be discontinued and the patient should be kept under close medical supervision.

■ Hematologic Effects

Leukopenia (white blood cell [WBC] count around 3500 mm^3) is fairly common, but not a clinically serious problem. If the WBC count is less than $3000/mm^3$ or the absolute neutrophil count (ANC) is less than $1000/mm^3$, the antipsychotic should be discontinued and the WBC should be monitored closely until it normalizes. Agranulocytosis is rare and reportedly occurs in 1/100,000 to 1/500,000 patients receiving traditional antipsychotics. It may occur most frequently with piperazine phenothiazines. The onset is usually within the first 3 months of therapy. If a patient develops signs and symptoms of infection, a WBC count with differential should be performed. Routine blood monitoring, however, is not indicated. Thrombocytopenia and pancytopenia have been reported to occur rarely.

■ Ophthalmic Side Effects

Secondary to anticholinergic effects of these medications, impairment in visual accommodation may result. This effect is usually temporary. Anticholinergic effects may also exacerbate narrow-angle glaucoma, which can result from increases in intraocular pressure. Higher-potency antipsychotics should be used in susceptible individuals.

Thioridazine is associated with irreversible pigmentation of the retina when given in doses greater than 800 mg/day. The pigmentation is caused by melanin deposits and is similar to retinitis pigmentosa, possibly progressing to blindness even following thioridazine discontinuation. Therefore, patients taking this medication should be monitored for this effect and the drug should be discontinued if any changes in pigmentation occur. Opaque whitish-brown deposits in the cornea and lens may occur with phenothiazine treatment, visible only by slit-lamp examination. They may progress to yellowish-brown granules, often stellate in shape. Although visual acuity is not usually affected, periodic slit-lamp ophthalmologic examinations are recommended in patients receiving long-term treatment with phenothiazines.

■ Dermatologic Effects

Allergic reactions rarely occur and do so primarily within the first 8 weeks of treatment. Rashes of maculopapular, petechial, erythematous, and urticarial manifestations have all been reported. Conventional antipsychotic drugs are often found in high concentrations in the skin of people taking them. A photosensitivity reaction that resembles a severe sunburn can occur in patients taking phenothiazines. This group of antipsychotics directly absorbs ultraviolet light and energy, resulting in the formation of free radicals, which can cause damage to the skin. Exposure to sunlight should be limited to between 30 and 60 minutes, and patients should be educated about the use of maximal blocking sunscreens, protective clothing, hats, and sunglasses.

Blue-gray to purplish skin discoloration, usually in areas of the body exposed to sunlight, can occur in patients receiving chlorpromazine. The coloration may begin as a tan or golden brown color and then progress to gray, blue, or purple tones. This generally occurs in patients:

- Receiving higher doses
- On long-term therapy
- Concurrently with a corneal or lens pigmentation.

■ Hepatic Effects

Abnormalities in liver function tests (LFTs), such as elevated aminotransferase and alkaline phosphatase, may occur in up to 50% of patients on conventional antipsychotics. Generally, these elevations occur without clinical significance, although they should be routinely monitored. If LFTs are elevated to greater than 3 times the upper limit of normal, the medication should be changed to a chemically unrelated agent.

Cholestatic hepatocellular jaundice occurs in approximately 2% of patients receiving phenothiazines, usually within the first 5 weeks of treatment. Prodromal symptoms often include:

- Malaise
- Fatigue
- Fever
- Chills
- Arthralgia
- Myalgia
- Gastrointestinal symptoms
- Severe pruritus.

The antipsychotic should be discontinued if jaundice occurs; once discontinued, symptoms usually disappear within 2 to 8 weeks. Pruritus may be palliatively treated with oral or topical antihistamines.

■ Epileptogenic Effects

Low-potency antipsychotic use may be associated with a slowing and an increased synchronization of the electroencephalogram (EEG). As a potential result, the lower-potency agents decrease the seizure threshold. Although this adverse effect is rare, administering a low-potency agent warrants consideration in patients with a seizure disorder or organic brain lesion.

■ Weight Gain

4

A common adverse effect of treatment with antipsychotics is weight gain, which can be significant in some cases. Weight gain may be mediated through blockade of the 5-hydroxytryptamine $(5\text{-}HT)_{2C}$ receptors as well as H_1. Average weight gain is between 1.5 kg and 6.9 kg (3.3 lb and 15.2 lb) over 6 months of treatment with conventional agents. Molindone and perhaps loxapine do not cause as great a weight gain as do the other antipsychotics. Patients should be educated about the morbidity associated with increases in weight such as:

- Hypercholesterolemia
- Diabetes
- Orthopedic complications
- Coronary artery disease.

Treatment plans should include diet modification and exercise, if possible. Weight gain is one of the primary reasons for noncompliance in patients taking conventional antipsychotics.

■ Endocrine Effects/Sexual Dysfunction

Antagonism of dopamine receptors in the tuberofundibular tract results in increased secretion of prolactin. The main physiologic effects of increased prolactin are suppression of gonadal activity and induction of the synthesis and secretion of milk. All conventional antipsychotics trigger a sustained increase in prolactin release. In men, the most commonly reported sexual dysfunctions are disturbances of erection and ejaculation, occurring in 30% to 60% of males treated with conventional antipsychotics. Women most likely experience decreased libido and orgasmic dysfunction, including difficulty achieving orgasm, changes in the quality of orgasm, and anorgasmia. This prevalence is slightly lower than in men, between 25% to 30%. Clinicians may not learn about these adverse effects if they do not ask about them specifically. Women may also experience menstrual irregularities, including amenorrhea and changes in the quantity of menses. Between 50% and 90% of women taking conventional antipsychotics experience some menstrual irregularity. Antagonism of alpha $(\alpha)_1$ receptors and anticholinergic effects may also contribute to sexual dysfunction. Treatment options include lowering the dosage or switching to an SGAD. Other drugs with anticholinergic properties should be discontinued. Bromocriptine, a dopamine agonist, has been used to improve libido in some patients in hyperprolactinemic states. Since other agents are available, eg, the SGADs, bromocriptine should generally not be used due to its ability to exacerbate psychoses and cause nausea and hypotension. Other endocrine side effects that may occur rarely include the inappropriate secretion of antidiuretic hormone and diabetes or impaired glucose tolerance.

■ Neuroleptic Malignant Syndrome

Neuroleptic malignant syndrome (NMS) is a life-threatening adverse effect of antipsychotic treatment. Mortality in well-developed cases ranges from 20% to 30%, although it may be much less according to recent studies. The clinical presentation of NMS evolves over 24 hours to 72 hours and usually includes:

- Severe muscular rigidity
- Autonomic instability:
  - Hyperthermia

- Tachycardia
  - Increased blood pressure
  - Tachypnea
  - Diaphoresis
- Altered consciousness.

A patient with NMS usually presents with muscle rigidity that progresses to include an elevated temperature, fluctuating consciousness, and unstable vital signs. These symptoms are often associated with elevations in creatine phosphokinase. Liver transaminase elevations, myoglobinemia, myoglobinuria, and leukocytosis may occur, as well as renal failure. Early symptoms of agitation may be mistaken for increased psychosis. Levenson's diagnostic criteria, the most accepted in the field, are listed in Table 4.6. For purposes of diagnosis, the patient should have two major manifestations and four minor manifestations, with a clinical history suggestive of the possibility of NMS.

TABLE 4.6 — LEVENSON'S DIAGNOSTIC CRITERIA FOR NEUROLEPTIC MALIGNANT SYNDROME
Major Manifestations • Fever • Rigidity • Elevated creatine phosphokinase
Minor Manifestations • Tachycardia • Abnormal blood pressure • Tachypnea • Altered consciousness • Diaphoresis • Leukocytosis

Rapid dose escalation and the use of high-potency antipsychotics at higher doses are associated with a greater incidence of NMS. Younger age, dehydration, previous episodes of NMS, and male gender are also risk factors for the development of NMS. The diagnosis is often difficult to discern and may result as an exclusion from many other possibilities. Patients present quite differently and may not experience all of the hallmark signs and symptoms. Other possible causative conditions should be ruled out by differential diagnosis (Table 4.7).

TABLE 4.7 — DIFFERENTIAL DIAGNOSIS FOR NEUROLEPTIC MALIGNANT SYNDROME
• Malignant hyperthermia • Lethal catatonia • Heat stroke • Severe extrapyramidal symptoms • Parkinson's disease • Central nervous system infection • Allergic drug reactions • Anticholinergic delirium • Systemic infection • Lithium toxicity

When NMS is diagnosed or suspected, antipsychotics should be discontinued and supportive and symptomatic treatment begun. This may include antipyretics, cooling blanket, intravenous fluids, oxygen, and adequate nutritional support. If a patient has a temperature greater than 101° F, treatment with dopamine agonists, such as bromocriptine, should be considered. The dose of bromocriptine is 2.5 mg po every 8 hours, increasing to a maximum of 60 mg/day. This should be continued for 10 days after the resolution of symptoms, then tapered off gradually. If such treatment is inadequate, dantrolene can be administered at 60 mg po every 6 hours. Liver transaminases should be monitored during therapy. After symptoms have resolved, patients should be treated with a different antipsychotic agent, avoiding high-potency and depot agents, if possible.

Use During Pregnancy and Lactation

The risk of teratogenesis with traditional antipsychotics is not well studied; however, its occurrence appears to be relatively low with the high-potency drugs. Haloperidol was once studied in the treatment of hyperemesis gravidarum without negative effects. Low-potency agents may be associated with a small increase in the relative risk for congenital anomalies. Altshuler and associates (1996) performed a meta-analysis of the effects of first-trimester exposure to low-potency antipsychotics and reported a baseline incidence of 2% increasing to 2.4% with treatment. Case reports have described limb malformations, but they appear to be rare. The risks of antipsychotic use must be weighed against the benefits of treatment. Clinicians may consider discontinuing antipsychotic drugs during the first trimester, but psychotic relapse in the mother can also be dangerous to the fetus. Antipsychotics are found in breast milk with the milk-to-plasma ratio of 0.5 to 1. Mothers who are being treated with traditional antipsychotics should receive a recommendation not to breast feed.

SUGGESTED READING

Altshuler LL, Cohen L, Szuba MP, Burt VK, Gitlin M, Mintz J. Pharmacologic management of psychiatric illness during pregnancy: dilemmas and guidelines. *Am J Psychiatry.* 1996;153:592-606.

McEvoy JP, Hogarty GE, Steingard S. Optimal dose of neuroleptic in acute schizophrenia. A controlled study of the neuroleptic threshold and higher haloperidol dose. *Arch Gen Psychiatry.* 1991; 48:739-745.

Schooler NR, Keith SJ, Severe JB, et al. Relapse and rehospitalization during maintenance treatment of schizophrenia. The effects of dose reduction and family treatment. *Arch Gen Psychiatry.* 1997;54:453-463.

Tandon R, Milner K, Jibson MD. Antipsychotics from theory to practice: integrating clinical and basic data. *J Clin Psychiatry.* 1999;60(suppl 8):21-28.

5

Extrapyramidal Symptoms/ Tardive Dyskinesia

Extrapyramidal symptoms (EPS), including akathisia, dystonia, and pseudoparkinsonism, are the major adverse effects associated with traditional antipsychotic therapy. These side effects are a result of dopamine antagonism in the nigrostriatal pathway. The rates of EPS with second-generation antipsychotic drugs (SGADs) are listed in Chapter 3, *Second-Generation Antipsychotic Drugs*.

5

Akathisia

Akathisia is the most frequently occurring of these adverse effects. Approximately 50% of patients treated with traditional agents will experience a subjective feeling of restlessness. These patients may pace, rock from foot to foot while standing, tap their feet, or move their feet restlessly while sitting. Frequently, patients complain that they are unable to feel comfortable regardless of what they do. Patients may feel anxious and irritable. Severe akathisia has resulted in aggressive and suicidal acts. The onset of akathisia is usually 5 to 10 days after the first dose or increase in dosage. Younger patients and those taking high doses of high-potency antipsychotics are at greater risk for the development of akathisia. This adverse effect may be difficult to diagnose and may be confused with anxiety, agitation, tardive dyskinesia, or a worsening of psychosis. The management of akathisia includes

- Reducing the antipsychotic dose
- Changing to another agent

- Use of lipid-soluble beta-blocking agents or benzodiazepines.

Propranolol, between 30 mg/day and 120 mg/day is highly effective for treatment, and relief is usually observed within 48 hours. Lorazepam (1 mg/day to 3 mg/day) and clonazepam (1 mg/day to 3 mg/day) may also be used for the treatment of akathisia. In general, SGADs cause less of this troubling side effect, but risperidone and olanzapine may be associated with this problem.

Dystonia

Acute dystonic reactions are abrupt in onset and are usually seen within 24 hours to 96 hours after a first dose or increase in dosage. Characteristic signs and symptoms may occur in 10% to 20% of patients and include abnormal positioning or spasm of the muscles of the head, neck, limbs, or trunk. Table 5.1 lists several forms of dystonia that may occur.

Risk factors for dystonia include:

- Young age
- African American race
- Patients with a history of acute dystonic reactions.

Dystonia almost always responds rapidly to antiparkinsonian medications and can usually be prevented either by pretreatment with these drugs or by limiting the neuroleptic dosage prescribed. Benztropine, 2 mg intramuscularly (IM), or diphenhydramine, 50 mg IM, will usually control the dystonia in 15 minutes to 20 minutes. Response to oral administration of these agents will not occur for 30 minutes to 40 minutes. If the initial dose does not provide control, another dose can be given in 30 minutes. Oral pro-

TABLE 5.1 — FORMS OF DYSTONIA	
Form of Dystonia	**Signs and Symptoms**
Blepharospasm	Involuntary tight contraction of the eyelids
Dysarthria	Unclear pronunciation or speech
Dysphagia	Difficulty in swallowing
Grimacing	Spasms of facial and jaw muscles
Macroglossia	Thickened or slurred speech due to hypertonic or enlarged tongue
Oculogyric crisis	Eyes deviated upward, downward, or sideways
Opisthotonos	Arching backward of the head, neck, and spine
Pharyngeal/laryngeal dystonia	Spasm of the throat, difficulty breathing
Tongue protrusion/ glossospasm	Spastic movements of the tongue
Torticollis/retrocollis	Abnormal positioning of the head and neck in relation to the rest of body
Trismus	Spasm of the jaw muscles, keeping the jaws tightly closed

phylaxis may include any of the anticholinergic medications listed in Table 5.2. If prophylaxis is used in a high-risk patient, its use should be reevaluated once the patient is stabilized on the antipsychotic. The incidence of dystonia is much less with the SGADs, but dystonic reactions have been reported with risperidone and olanzapine.

TABLE 5.2 — DOSING RANGES FOR ANTICHOLINERGICS	
Generic (Trade) Name	**Usual Dose Range**
Amantadine (Symmetrel)	100 mg bid-tid
Benztropine (Cogentin)	1-2 mg bid
Biperiden (Akineton)	1-3 mg bid
Diphenhydramine (Benadryl)	25-50 mg bid
Orphenadrine (Norflex)	100 mg bid
Procyclidine (Kemedrine)	2.5-5 mg tid
Trihexyphenidyl (Artane)	1-3 mg tid

Pseudoparkinsonism

Pseudoparkinsonism resembles idiopathic Parkinson's disease and occurs in approximately 15% of patients treated with traditional antipsychotics. The onset of symptoms is usually seen within 1 to 2 weeks following initiation or a dose increase. Risk factors include:

- Older age
- Female gender
- High doses
- Possibly those with depressive symptoms.

A patient may have any of the four cardinal symptoms listed in Table 5.3.

The management of pseudoparkinsonism includes a dose reduction, switching to a different agent, or the use of anticholinergic or dopaminergic drugs. Any of the anticholinergic agents listed in the Table 5.2 are effective for relieving parkinsonlike symptoms. Benztropine has a longer half-life, thus allowing twice-daily dosing. Trihexyphenidyl has more abuse potential, whereas diphenhydramine produces more

TABLE 5.3 — CARDINAL SYMPTOMS OF PSEUDOPARKINSONISM

- Akinesia, bradykinesia, or decreased motor activity including difficulty initiating movement and extreme slowness, masklike facial expression, micrographia, slowed speech, and decreased arm swing
- Tremor, known as pill-rolling type, predominant at rest, decreases with movement, usually involves the fingers and hands, although it may be seen in the arms, legs, neck, head, and chin (it may often be activated by having the patient perform mechanical movements with one extremity, 4 to 7 cycles/sec)
- Cogwheel rigidity, seen as the patient's limbs yield in jerky, rachetlike fashion when passively moved by the examiner (a mild form may present as stiffness)
- Postural abnormalities and instability manifested as stooped posture, difficulty in maintaining stability when changing body position, and a gait that ranges from slow and shuffling to festinating (a result of dysfunction in autonomic stability combined with a shift in the center of gravity due to the stooped posture)

sedation than the other agents. With all of these treatments, symptoms will usually resolve in 3 to 4 days, but a minimum of at least 2 weeks of treatment is normally required for complete response. Amantadine is as effective as anticholinergic agents, with significantly less effect on memory function. Dosage adjustment is necessary with renal insufficiency and livedo reticularis may occur in 1% to 5% of patients. Some patients may experience a reduction in benefit after 1 to 3 months of amantadine treatment.

Tardive Dyskinesia

■ Epidemiology

Tardive dyskinesia (TD) is a syndrome characterized by abnormal choreiform (rapid, objectively, purposeless, irregular, and spontaneous) and athetoid (slow and irregular) movements occurring late in onset in relation to initiation of antipsychotic therapy. This adverse effect usually develops over several months and occurs after at least 3 months of conventional antipsychotic treatment. The estimated average prevalence is 20%, with a range of 13% to 36%. The incidence of new cases per treatment year is approximately 5%. The incidence with SGADs is less than 2%. TD is reversible in one third to one half of cases with the cessation of the antipsychotic. When the antipsychotic is tapered or discontinued, there is usually worsening of abnormal movements initially. Risk factors include:

- Older age
- Duration of antipsychotic treatment
- Higher rates of EPS
- Substance abuse
- Mood disorders.

■ Signs and Symptoms

The characteristic signs and symptoms usually involve a buccolingual-masticatory syndrome or orofacial movements. Typically, these are the first detectable signs of TD and can progress to movements severe enough to interfere with chewing, speech, respiration, or swallowing. These include:

- Lip smacking
- Puckering
- Sucking
- Pouting
- Tongue writhing, protrusion, and tremor.

Other facial movements include frequent blinking, grimacing, and tics. Truncal and limb movements usually are seen as TD progresses. This includes twisting, spreading, flexion, and extension of the fingers and toe dorsiflexion. Unusual posture, hyperextension, pelvic thrusting, exaggerated lordosis (bending backward), rocking, and swaying may all occur in the truncal area. While younger adults report more truncal movements, older patients experience more orofacial movements. Voluntary attempts to suppress the movements usually work temporarily but may actually lead to worsening of the symptoms.

■ Pathophysiology

The pathophysiology of TD is complex and has not been satisfactorily explained. The original theory involves dopamine supersensitivity of striatal dopamine receptors due to long-term antipsychotic treatment. This, however, does not entirely explain the pathogenesis of TD. This may partially be true, but depletion of gamma-aminobutyric acid (GABA) may also play a role. Decreased GABA turnover or binding sites may occur after chronic antipsychotic exposure, leading to increased inhibition of GABAergic outflow. This results in a loss of inhibition to the thalamocortical projections. Increased activity may lead to blockade of dopamine $(D)_2$ projections. Other neurotransmitters and neuropeptides may play a role in the etiology such as cholecystokinin, and changes at the *N*-methyl-D-aspartate (NMDA) and opiate receptors may be involved.

■ Treatment

Dosage reduction may decrease or eliminate symptoms in some patients. However, the development of TD is a medical, legal, and ethical problem. If patients with TD are kept on antipsychotic therapy, there is the possibility of symptoms worsening. Prevention of this adverse effect is important. Patients with clear target symptoms should be treated at the minimum effective dose. Regular examinations and assessments should be done to ensure that patients do not have signs and symptoms. Switching to or initiating therapy with an SGAD may prevent TD, since these drugs appear to have a lower incidence of this problem. Minimizing the use of anticholinergics is also important. There are no Food and Drug Administration-approved agents for the treatment of TD. Many therapies have been tried with little success. Benzodiazepines, such as clonazepam, are sometimes initially effective but usually lose efficacy by 3 to 4 months. Valproate and baclofen have also been used with modest results. Dopamine-depleting agents, such as reserpine and methyldopa, may alleviate symptoms in some patients but have many serious side effects associated with their use. Calcium channel blockers and botulinus toxin have also been tried with little positive effects. Vitamin E has been tried in several double-blind trials with mixed results. The dose range usually used is 1200 IU to 1600 IU for 4 to 12 weeks. Vitamin E may be more effective in patients who have had TD for less than 5 years. Nonetheless, the beneficial effects of vitamin E are modest.

Clozapine may be effective in ameliorating existing TD. Patients with moderate to severe TD will usually have marked improvements in their symptoms when changed to clozapine from conventional antipsychotics. However, approximately 9 months to 10 months of clozapine treatment may be required before the effects of TD begin to remit. The American Psychiatric Association Task Force on Tardive Dyskinesia (1992) has issued recommendations for the prevention and management of TD (Table 5.4).

TABLE 5.4 — PREVENTION AND MANAGEMENT OF TARDIVE DYSKINESIA

- Establish objective evidence that antipsychotic medications are effective for an individual
- Use the lowest effective dose of antipsychotic
- Prescribe cautiously to children, elderly people, and individuals with mood disorders
- Examine patients on a regular basis for evidence of tardive dyskinesia
- When tardive dyskinesia is diagnosed, consider alternatives to antipsychotics, obtain informed consent, and also consider dosage reduction
- If the tardive dyskinesia worsens, consider a number of options, including discontinuing the antipsychotics, switching to a different drug, or initiating a trial of clozapine

SUGGESTED READING

Akiyama K. Algorithms for neuroleptic-associated tardive movement disorders. *Psychiatry Clin Neurosci*. 1999;53(suppl):S23-S29.

Casey DE. Effects of clozapine therapy in schizophrenic individuals at risk for tardive dyskinesia. *J Clin Psychiatry*. 1998;59(suppl 3):31-37.

Casey DE. Tardive dyskinesia and atypical antipsychotic drugs. *Schizophr Res*. 1999;35(suppl):S61-S66.

Collaborative Working Group on Clinical Trial Evaluations. Assessment of EPS and tardive dyskinesia in clinical trials. *J Clin Psychiatry*. 1998;59(suppl 12):23-27.

Gerlach J. The continuing problem of extrapyramidal symptoms: strategies for avoidance and effective treatment. *J Clin Psychiatry*. 1999;60(suppl 23):20-24.

Gupta S, Mosnik D, Black DW, Berry S, Masand PS. Tardive dyskinesia: review of treatments past, present, and future. *Ann Clin Psychiatry*. 1999;11:257-266.

Lader M. Some adverse effects of antipsychotics: prevention and treatment. *J Clin Psychiatry*. 1999;60(suppl 12):18-21.

Van Putten T, Marder SR. Behavioral toxicity of antipsychotic drugs. *J Clin Psychiatry*. 1987;48(suppl):13-19.

6

Management of Acute Psychosis, Psychiatric Emergencies, and Aggressive/Suicidal Behavior

Psychiatric Emergencies and Acute Psychosis

6

Psychiatric emergencies are often found in the emergency departments but may also occur in the psychiatric unit, in a medical facility, or in the outpatient setting. Most psychiatric emergencies require both pharmacologic and psychotherapeutic intervention. Often the psychiatrist must make decisions based on limited information or history. Each state has a statute that requires a physician to detain patients involuntarily in a psychiatric facility if the patient is judged to be dangerous to self or others. Patients who do not take care of their physical needs secondary to their psychosis, but are nonviolent, may still represent a threat to themselves or others, but this decision is often based on clinical judgment. Psychiatric patients who are considered dangerous may be legally detained and treated against their will; however, in most states, they cannot be chronically medicated without their consent unless a court order is obtained.

The two medications most often used for acute agitation are lorazepam and haloperidol. Either of these drugs can be given intravenously but are generally given by intramuscular (IM) injection (Table 6.1). Either medication is useful in ameliorating acute psychosis. Lorazepam is much better tolerated by patients than haloperidol. This is crucial, since patients will tend to resist the use of lorazepam much less than haloperidol, further enhancing its usefulness in acute care.

TABLE 6.1 — DOSES OF MEDICATIONS FOR PSYCHIATRIC EMERGENCIES AND ACUTE PSYCHOSIS	
Drug	**Dose**
Lorazepam (Ativan)	1-2 mg IM q hour prn
Haloperidol (Haldol)	5-10 mg IM twice daily

Chlorpromazine and diazepam IM injections have also been used, although diazepam is erratically absorbed from the deltoid muscle and chlorpromazine is associated with marked orthostatic hypotension and burning upon injection. Haloperidol may cause extrapyramidal symptoms (EPS), such as dystonic reactions, that can be particularly distressing and an experience like this may cause the patient to avoid acute care. Haloperidol and chlorpromazine injections are more bioavailable than when the drugs are given orally; thus higher doses will reach systemic circulation better with injections than orally. Haloperidol is about 50% bioavailable; thus 10 mg orally is equivalent to a 5-mg IM injection. Chlorpromazine is about 25% bioavailable, with 100 mg orally being similar to 25 mg by IM injection. When EPS occur, anticholinergic agents should be given parenterally (see Chapter 5, *Extrapyramidal Symptoms/Tardive Dyskinesia*).

Treatment for acute schizophrenic exacerbation has changed in the past decade. Rapid tranquilization (neuroleptization) with antipsychotics, such as haloperidol in 5-mg doses administered every hour as needed, has been replaced by 10 mg/day to 20 mg/day of haloperidol or the acute use of second-generation antipsychotic drugs (SGADs) in combination with a benzodiazepine (usually lorazepam) as needed. Benzodiazepine augmentation of antipsychotics has been shown to control agitation during exacerbations of schizophrenia.

Aggressive Behavior

Between 10% and 12% of patients with schizophrenia or major affective disorder may exhibit violent or aggressive behavior. Persistent, overt physical aggression is dangerous to both the victims and the perpetrators. In clinical practice, aggressive patients have often been treated with higher doses of antipsychotic medications, but this therapeutic approach has not been proven effective. In fact, higher doses may cause akathisia and irritability that may lead to increased aggressive behavior. Other pharmacologic strategies that have been used with varying results include anticonvulsants, benzodiazepines, serotonin reuptake inhibitors, and beta-blocking agents. Additionally, some medications may cause aggressive behavior. Table 6.2 lists medications that have been linked to aggressive behavior.

TABLE 6.2 — MEDICATIONS LINKED TO AGGRESSIVE BEHAVIOR

Drug Class	Specific Agents
Sedatives/anxiolytics	Alcohol, benzodiazepines, sedative anticonvulsants (eg, phenobarbital)
Stimulants	Cocaine, amphetamines, phenylpropanolamine
Antidepressants	Tricyclics, fluoxetine, fluvoxamine
Miscellaneous	Marijuana, anabolic steroids

The SGADs have been shown to decrease some aggressive behavior. Several open, uncontrolled studies have demonstrated the antiaggressive effects of clozapine. These effects on aggressive behavior may be specific in that they are not mediated by sedation and are relatively independent of its general antipsychotic effect. Studies have found clozapine to decrease violent episodes, decrease the need for seclusion, and decrease hostility as measured by Brief Psychiatric Rating Scale (BPRS) hostility scores. Clozapine patients demonstrated the antiaggressive effects within 6 months of initiation, with some cases becoming less aggressive during the first few weeks. A few controlled clinical trials have examined risperidone vs conventional antipsychotics or placebo in regard to hostility as measured by these items on the BPRS or Positive and Negative Syndrome Scale. Risperidone has been shown to be superior to placebo and appears to offer benefits compared with conventional antipsychotics. Risperidone has been found to exert this effect independent of other symptoms. Several open reports have shown decreases in the need for seclusion and restraints as well. Quetiapine and olanzapine may offer benefits as well but have been reported only sparsely in the literature. Of the antipsychotics currently available, clozapine may offer the most benefits in patients who are persistently aggressive, and risperidone may be the best overall choice for routine chronic use.

Treatment of Suicidal Behavior

Suicide is the chief cause of premature death in individuals with schizophrenia. Between 20% and 40% of schizophrenic patients will attempt suicide at some point in their lifetime, and approximately 10% will die by this means. Risk factors identified in patients with schizophrenia are listed in Table 6.3.

In conjunction with other treatments, antipsychotic medications are commonly used to decrease the risk of suicide in patients with schizophrenia. Although there has been much inconsistency in the lit-

TABLE 6.3 — RISK FACTORS FOR SUICIDE IN PEOPLE WITH SCHIZOPHRENIA	
Category	**Risk Factor**
Gender	Male
Race	White
Marital status	Never married, divorced, or widowed
Suicide history	Family history of suicide, history of suicide attempts
Intelligence	Relatively high intelligence quotient
Vocational history	Unemployed, early vocational difficulties, poor work functioning
Social support	Social isolation, limited external support
Substance-abuse history	Current or past substance abuse, especially alcohol
Depressive symptoms	Significant depressive symptoms or mood, depressive episode at last psychiatric visit, sense of hopelessness, hostility, depression, paranoid ideation, obsessive-compulsiveness, hospitalization for which a depressive episode was part of diagnosis
Psychotic symptoms	Command hallucinations, negative association with positive symptoms
Awareness of illness	Fear of further mental deterioration, awareness of deteriorative effects of schizophrenia
Course of illness	Frequent hospitalizations, recent discharge, acute exacerbations, worsening disease trend, frequent relapses and rehospitalizations, high post-discharge levels of psychopathology and functional impairment
Length of illness	Shorter duration of illness
Medication	Not receiving antipsychotics or relatively low or high antipsychotic doses

6

erature pertaining to conventional agents and suicide risk, treatment with recommended doses of these agents may be effective in decreasing suicidality. However, patients on extremely low or high doses have been found to have a higher likelihood of committing suicide. This is most likely due to EPS (particularly akathisia) and tardive dyskinesia (TD) at higher doses and lack of efficacy at lower doses.

Several studies have examined clozapine and its effect on suicidality. Clozapine has been found to reduce the rate of suicide attempts as well as decrease the seriousness and lethality of attempts. Mortality rates have been found to be lower during clozapine use than during periods without its use. Clozapine may provide benefits by its ability to treat TD, positive symptoms, and depressive symptoms without producing EPS. Additionally, there is extensive evidence that diminished serotoninergic activity may be related to suicide. Both animal and clinical studies have shown that a reduction in central serotonin function appears to be associated with suicidal, parasuicidal, and impulsive-aggressive behavior. The reduction by clozapine of suicide risk in schizophrenic patients is consistent with its reported antidepressant effects, which are achieved, in part, by normalization of serotoninergic function. The release of serotonin in the prefrontal cortex is seen with long-term clozapine therapy. The other SGADs have not yet been reported effective for decreasing suicidality. Risperidone, olanzapine, and quetiapine may be beneficial due to their lower side effect profiles and their effect on serotonin. Studies with these new agents are needed in this important area.

SUGGESTED READING

Buckley PF. The role of typical and atypical antipsychotic medications in the management of agitation and aggression. *J Clin Psychiatry*. 1999;60(suppl 10):52-60.

Harkavy-Friedman JM, Nelson E. Management of the suicidal patient with schizophrenia. *Psychiatr Clin North Am*. 1997;20:625-640.

Kane JM. Pharmacologic treatment of schizophrenia. *Biol Psychiatry*. 1999;46:1396-1408.

Meltzer HY. Suicide in schizophrenia: risk factors and clozapine treatment. *J Clin Psychiatry*. 1998;59(suppl 3):15-20.

Palmer DD, Henter ID, Wyatt RJ. Do antipsychotic medications decrease the risk of suicide in patients with schizophrenia? *J Clin Psychiatry*. 1999;60(suppl 2):100-103.

Radomsky ED, Haas GL, Mann JJ, Sweeney JA. Suicidal behavior in patients with schizophrenia and other psychotic disorders. *Am J Psychiatry*. 1999;156:1590-1595.

Schatzberg AF, De Battista C. Phenomenology and treatment of agitation. *J Clin Psychiatry*. 1999;60(suppl 15):17-20.

Steinert T, Wiebe C, Gebhardt RP. Aggressive behavior against self and others among first-admission patients with schizophrenia. *Psychiatr Serv*. 1999;50:85-90.

Volavka J, Citrome L. Atypical antipsychotics in the treatment of the persistently aggressive psychotic patient: methodological concerns. *Schizophr Res*. 1999;35(suppl):S23-S33.

7 Continuation and Maintenance Therapy With Antipsychotics

Stabilization and Maintenance Therapy

If a patient has improved on a particular antipsychotic medication or medication regimen, the patient should continue to receive this same therapy at the same dose for the next 6 months before a lower maintenance dose is considered for continued treatment. Premature lowering of the dose or discontinuation of the medication during this phase may lead to relatively rapid relapse. Patients who have been stable for over 6 months and have no positive symptoms may be candidates for a dose reduction. This should be done gradually and to no less than at least one fifth of the usual maintenance dose as long as the patient remains stable.

Reviewing the need for maintenance antipsychotic medication should be done at least annually. Patients who have had no or very few symptoms throughout the year of maintenance treatment should be considered for a trial period without medication. Once this decision is made, the medication should be tapered slowly and gradually over many months. More frequent monitoring or visits are recommended and the use of early intervention strategies such as education about early symptoms is important during this time. In patients who experience multiple episodes of symptoms, maintenance therapy should be continued for at least 5 years and probably indefinitely. The use of antipsychotics should continue in patients with suicidal or aggressive behavior. The long-term benefits of continuous antipsychotic medications are still not well understood because of the side effects and low compliance with conventional agents. Long-term studies of second-generation antipsychotic drugs suggest that benefits of these agents may accumulate over years of continued use.

Compliance

People with schizophrenia are often known to be noncompliant with medication. Factors that contribute to noncompliance with therapy include:

- Side effects
- Lack of insight
- Belief that the medication is ineffective.

Specific factors have predicted higher rates of noncompliance (Table 7.1). Older, grandiose, substance-abusing, and deficit patients have more difficulty with compliance. Compliance is difficult to quantify, measure, and study because compliance is rarely an all-or-none phenomenon, but may include mistakes in dosing, timing, omitting doses, or taking medications that are not prescribed. Estimates of noncompliance range from approximately 24% to 88%, with a mean of approximately 50% of people with schizophrenia who are noncompliant with prescribed therapy. Patients who are noncompliant have approximately a 4-fold greater risk of relapse than those who are compliant. Physicians often overestimate the compliance of their patients, which, in turn, does not allow them to consider noncompliance as a likely explanation for treatment failures.

Between 25% and 66% of patients who discontinue prescribed antipsychotic therapy cited adverse effects as the primary reason for noncompliance. Both self and physician ratings of side effects are associ-

TABLE 7.1 — FACTORS RELATED TO COMPLIANCE
Patient-Related Factors • Greater illness severity or grandiosity • Lack of insight • Substance abuse comorbidity
Medication-Related Factors • Dysphoric medication side effects • Subtherapeutic or excessively high doses
Environmental Factors • Inadequate support or supervision • Practical barriers, such as lack of money or transportation
Clinician-Related Factors • Poor therapeutic alliance
Adapted from: Fenton WS, et al. *Schizophr Bull.* 1997;23:637-651.

7

ated with higher rates of noncompliance. Extrapyramidal symptoms, most notably akathisia, sexual dysfunction, and weight gain, are the adverse effects that lead to the greatest noncompliance. SGADs are associated with better rates of compliance, which is most likely attributable to better side effect profiles. This leads to lowering rates of relapse and rehospitalization, improving patient care, and reducing overall costs (see Chapter 12, *Outcomes and Health-Services Research*). A good relationship between the patient and the physician is important to establish rapport and trust, the groundwork for enhancing a patient's acceptance of the therapy. Patient and family education, including expectations and potential adverse effects, is important. The emergence of adverse events should be taken seriously and treated immediately.

SUGGESTED READING

Fenton WS, Blyler CR, Heinssen RK. Determinants of medication compliance in schizophrenia: empirical and clinical findings. *Schizophr Bull.* 1997;23:637-651.

Hogarty GE, Ulrich RF. The limitations of antipsychotic medication on schizophrenia relapse and adjustment and the contributions of psychosocial treatment. *J Psychiatr Res*. 1998;32:243-250.

Marder SR. Antipsychotic drugs and relapse prevention. *Schizophr Res*. 1999;35(suppl):S87-S92.

Robinson D, Woerner MG, Alvir JM, et al. Predictors of relapse following response from a first episode of schizophrenia or schizoaffective disorder. *Arch Gen Psychiatry.* 1999;56:241-247.

8 Treatment-Resistant Schizophrenia

One fifth to one third of all cases of schizophrenia are resistant to drug treatment. These patients are highly symptomatic and require extensive periods of hospital care. There has been a great deal of excitement following the demonstration of clozapine's efficacy in inpatients with treatment-resistant schizophrenia. However, clozapine treatment carries with it significant morbidity, including:

- Serious side effects
- Need for ongoing weekly blood monitoring
- High cost.

Many clinicians and patients hoped that other new antipsychotics would share clozapine's effectiveness without its most serious side effects. However, no other antipsychotic has clozapine's efficacy in this patient group. The incidence of resistance to antipsychotic therapy and thus the need for clozapine in such patients is lessened by optimal use of second-generation and depot antipsychotics.

Chronicity vs Treatment Resistance

Commonly, treatment resistance has been considered to be roughly equivalent to chronic or frequent hospitalization. This is not an adequate definition. Patients should also have current and persistent positive symptoms of psychosis and at least moderate overall severity of illness in order for nonresponsiveness to apply, as chronic hospitalization can occur despite low levels of symptoms.

Many people with schizophrenia who have been chronically hospitalized may not be truly resistant to drug treatment. Inadequate psychosocial programming, poor compliance with prescribed drug therapy, and a history of committing violence are all risk factors for chronic hospitalization. Therefore, an optimized medication and treatment trial should be employed before a patient's illness is considered nonresponsive. In addition, both the effects of drug noncompliance and extrapyramidal symptoms (EPS) can mimic true treatment resistance. At least a 1- to 2-year course of persistent symptoms should also be considered one of the criteria for treatment resistance in schizophrenia because of the waxing and waning course of this illness.

Definition of Treatment Resistance

The most accepted current criteria for treatment resistance in schizophrenia were first widely used by Kane and associates. These criteria, modified for clinical use, are presented in Table 8.1.

Defining Adequate Drug Trials

Two retrospective drug trial failures are as effective as three in screening for treatment resistance. People not responsive to two adequate antipsychotic trials (one retrospective and one prospective) have less than a 7% chance of responding to another trial. The Food and Drug Administration (FDA) guidelines for clozapine's use, as reflected in the product labeling for Clozaril, also state that people should fail to respond to two separate trials of antipsychotics before being treated with clozapine.

It is generally recognized that a 4- to 6-week period (rather than strictly a 6-week period) is adequate for a treatment trial of an antipsychotic. Doses of

TABLE 8.1 — CRITERIA FOR TREATMENT RESISTANCE IN SCHIZOPHRENIA

- Persistent positive psychotic symptoms of at least two of four common positive symptoms:
  - Hallucinatory behavior
  - Suspiciousness
  - Unusual thought content
  - Conceptual disorganization
- Current presence of at least a moderately severe illness
- Persistence of illness: no period of good social and/or occupational functioning within the past 5 years
- Drug-refractory condition defined as at least two periods of treatment within the preceding 5 years with appropriate doses of conventional or second-generation antipsychotics, each without clinically significant symptom relief

greater than or equal to 400 mg/day of chlorpromazine have been shown to be adequate to block 80% to 90% of dopamine receptors (thought to be the target of this drug action). Higher doses produce no direct therapeutic benefit, even in patients not responsive to therapy, and do not have greater efficacy than lower doses in acute treatment. Therefore, two 4- to 6-week trials of 400 mg to 600 mg chlorpromazine are now accepted as a standard for an adequate trial.

Neurobiology of Treatment Resistance in Schizophrenia

Until the arrival of standardized criteria for defining treatment resistance, research into the neurobiologic nature of the problem had been scant. Recently, however, with the use of more objective criteria, some consistent findings have been seen. There is a relative paucity of data in this area, and more research needs to be done. People with treatment-resistant schizophrenia appear to have increased cortical atrophy on magnetic resonance imaging (MRI) compared with those with responsive illness. This is particularly true if they have predominant negative symptoms.

Lack of response to early treatment is also predictive of nonresponse. The most intriguing finding about predicting which new drugs may be effective in treatment-resistant schizophrenia has been the fact that such people appear to have lower catecholamine levels in the cerebrospinal fluid (CSF). Clozapine response has been associated with low ratios of CSF homovanillic acid to 5-hydroxyindoleacetic acid. These findings suggest that drugs with low dopamine antagonism and high serotoninergic antagonism may be particularly useful in treatment-resistant schizophrenia.

Drug Therapy for Treatment Resistance

Historically, drug therapy for treatment-resistant schizophrenia centered either on the use of different dose strategies of conventional antipsychotics or on the use of adjunct agents such as lithium, beta-blocking drugs, anticonvulsants, and benzodiazepines. Since the arrival of clozapine, attention in the field has shifted to a greater focus on the use of new antipsychotics for treatment resistance in schizophrenia. This interest has occurred because of the demonstration of the superior efficacy of clozapine and the fact that new antipsychotics must either have been shown to have significantly fewer side effects or improved efficacy compared with a conventional antipsychotic (usually haloperidol) in order to be marketed in the United States.

Conventional Antipsychotic Drugs

Conventional antipsychotic drugs have long been the first-line drug therapy for treating schizophrenia. In controlled trials of people with drug-resistant symptoms, fewer than 5% responded after having their drug therapy changed from one conventional antipsychotic to another. If no clinical improvement is seen after 2 weeks of therapy, compliance with medication should be evaluated. If the patient is compliant, a different drug trial should be considered after 4 weeks to 6 weeks of minimal response.

Second-Generation Antipsychotic Drugs

Second-generation antipsychotic drugs should be the first consideration after the failure of conventional drug therapy. These drugs are also effective as first-line therapy (with the exception of clozapine, because of its serious side effects). 8

■ Clozapine

Clozapine was approved for use by the FDA in 1990 specifically for the treatment of patients whose symptoms do not adequately respond to conventional antipsychotic therapy, either because therapy was not effective or because it could not be continued secondary to intolerable side effects. It is still the only drug with proven efficacy in rigorously defined treatment-resistant schizophrenia, and approximately 30% of treatment-refractory patients will respond to this medication. However, fewer than 8% of new antipsychotic prescriptions are written for clozapine. This phenomenon of relative under-usage probably relates to the cost and complexity of clozapine therapy. These arise from the need for long-term hematologic monitoring for agranulocytosis and persistent serious side effects, such as weight gain, sialorrhea, and sedation that can accompany therapy with clozapine.

The optimal dose strategy for clozapine is a slow dose escalation. Patients should be evaluated for response at dose plateaus of 200 mg/day to 400 mg/day and 500 mg/day to 600 mg/day. Only patients with few side effects to clozapine should be titrated to doses higher than 600 mg/day. Patients should not be titrated to a higher dose of clozapine if myoclonus is present, as this side effect may precede the development of seizures.

■ Risperidone

It is been widely recognized that risperidone treatment is usually not effective in clozapine responders who are treatment-resistant. Risperidone is more effective than conventional antipsychotics for positive and affective symptoms in patients with acute schizophrenia. Wirshing and others found a 24% response rate to risperidone as compared with an 11% response rate to haloperidol after 4 weeks in patients who were treatment-resistant. Although risperidone does not appear to be as effective as clozapine for treatment resistance, it may be worth a trial even after traditional antipsychotics have failed prior to using clozapine.

■ Olanzapine

Olanzapine is effective in treatment-responsive schizophrenia, with superiority in negative and affective symptoms in acute patients. It has a low incidence of EPS and is not different from placebo in its incidence of akathisia. It does not, however, have clozapine-like efficacy in well-characterized treatment resistance. Conley and others found only a 7% response rate in a treatment-refractory population. Additionally, 40% of those treatment failures went on to respond to clozapine.

■ **Quetiapine**

Quetiapine has been shown to be effective in treatment-responsive schizophrenia. There was no difference between placebo and quetiapine in the amount of EPS or akathisia in published trials to date. This drug is not more effective than haloperidol in acute schizophrenia, and there is no controlled trial of this agent in treatment resistance. This drug can be useful in patients who cannot tolerate the EPS of other antipsychotics.

Alternate Therapies

If patients remain refractory to treatment after trials of novel agents, alternate therapies should be considered. These include:

- Adjunct medication
- Reserpine
- Electroconvulsive therapy (ECT).

The data concerning the efficacy of these therapies are limited, but they may be of use in some patients.

■ **Lithium and Anticonvulsants**

Adjunct lithium therapy has been seen to be beneficial in some patients with treatment-resistant schizophrenia; however, these patients were often not defined by the rigorous criteria of later studies. These published trials of adjunct lithium which are positive, have been conducted with small numbers of patients, and often the criteria for defining treatment resistance were not clear or were overinclusive. More recent reports have found no benefits with adjunct lithium therapy and fluphenazine decanoate. Lithium should be used with caution in combination with conventional antipsychotics or clozapine because of the recognized dangers of delirium, encephalopathy, and neurotoxicity that have been reported with these combinations.

Carbamazepine and valproic acid have been observed to be effective in bipolar affective disorder and are often considered as adjunct therapy in patients with schizophrenia. However, trials involving these agents have had relatively few subjects. Positive effects seen with carbamazepine and valproate have been modest and usually involved nonspecific improvement in areas such as behavior and social adjustment. Carbamazepine should be used with caution due to reports of disorientation and ataxia associated with its use. It can also reduce the blood level of haloperidol by as much as 50%. Carbamazepine should not be used in combination with clozapine. There are few data with newer anticonvulsants, although a few positive results were seen with lamotrigine adjunctive treatment with clozapine.

■ Benzodiazepines

There have been several reports on the use of adjunct benzodiazepines in treatment-resistant schizophrenia. Results have been mixed, with some double-blind studies showing a treatment effect, while other studies are negative. Given that patients with schizophrenia frequently experience anxiety and irritability, it is not surprising that benzodiazepines often prove to be useful agents in the treatment of this disorder. There is no firm evidence for a specific adjunct antipsychotic effect with these agents, however. They should be used with caution because of the risks of chronic sedation, fatigue ataxia, and dependence. There are some reports of behavioral disinhibition with these drugs and the possibility of synergistic respiratory toxicity with clozapine.

■ Other Therapies

There are historical studies suggesting that beta-blockers and reserpine may be useful in refractory schizophrenia. However, there are no available controlled studies with current diagnostic criteria. There is limited evidence that long-term therapy with either of these strategies is beneficial. There have been no controlled studies of ECT to date in treatment-resistant schizophrenic patients. Before the use of clozapine, there was some evidence from uncontrolled trials that ECT provided benefit for treatment-resistant patients, but usually the effect of ECT has been the most robust in patients with an illness of short duration. There have been a few open trials of ECT in patients who had an inadequate clozapine response. These trials showed some benefit from ECT. However, issues of persistence of effect and long-term maintenance of these patients have not yet been addressed.

There are very few positive data available supporting the use of two antipsychotic medications. The introduction of another antipsychotic should only occur when optimization of all other treatments has failed. The concurrent use should be objectively rated for improvements in symptoms. If no significant improvements are seen, the second agent should be discontinued, since the risk for adverse effects outweighs the benefits.

Summary

A defined approach to patients with treatment-resistant schizophrenia is critical. The practices outlined in Table 8.2 should maximize the likelihood of a successful outcome for an antipsychotic drug trial for treatment resistance.

Since the antipsychotics being introduced today may have different mechanisms of action than conventional antipsychotics and than each other, clinicians will need to explore the possibility of response with each of these new agents in turn with their patients with persistently refractory symptoms. To date, clozapine

TABLE 8.2 — APPROACH TO PATIENTS WITH TREATMENT-RESISTANT SCHIZOPHRENIA
• Identification of defined target symptoms. Antipsychotics are most helpful for the positive symptoms of psychosis: hallucinations, delusions, and thought disorder. Newer medications may also be helpful in reducing negative symptoms, such as poor socialization, withdrawal and affective blunting, particularly if these are secondary to extrapyramidal symptoms of conventional antipsychotics. Clozapine has been shown to be effective in hostile, aggressive, psychotic patients. Understanding the target symptoms for a specific drug trial will allow for greater clarity in defining the parameters of success and failure. • The systematic use of drugs at sufficient dosages and for a sufficient duration to establish efficacy. This is particularly critical before adjunct drugs are used since these may complicate the therapeutic situation to the point where defining the optimal drug treatment for a patient is not possible. • Consideration that medication intolerance, noncompliance, inadequate social support, and inadequate psychosocial treatment may create the appearance of treatment resistance. A consideration of these factors should precede the declaration that any drug therapy is a failure. Although therapeutic ranges of most antipsychotics are not well established, measuring blood levels may be useful to establish compliance and to rule out the unlikely event of poor medication absorption. • Exhausting the utility of single agents before using multiple agents. There is tremendous pressure for the clinician to find a drug to rapidly treat every psychological problem manifest in a patient. It is important to remember that no adjunct agent has ever been shown to robustly improve antipsychotic response. Hostility, irritability, insomnia, and withdrawal can all be secondary to psychosis and may resolve only after a patient has experienced a good antipsychotic drug effect.

- Aggressively preventing extrapyramidal symptoms through the appropriate choice of primary therapy. With the arrival of antipsychotic agents that are clearly effective at doses that do not produce extrapyramidal symptoms in the vast majority of patients, we should be able to almost eliminate persistent side effects as a reason for therapeutic failure.
- Maintaining a positive therapeutic attitude. There are more choices now for antipsychotic therapy than ever before, with new drugs appearing annually. Patients should be encouraged to think that there is good reason to be optimistic that some therapy will be found that will be beneficial to them, even if they have had a history of severe illness.

is the only medication with demonstrated efficacy in treatment resistance. The differential efficacy of new drugs in treatment-resistant schizophrenia will only be clear when well-designed double-blind studies using rigorous entry criteria are completed.

SUGGESTED READING

Bustillo JR, Lauriello J, Keith SJ. Schizophrenia: improving outcome. *Harv Rev Psychiatry.* 1999;6:229-240.

Conley RR, Buchanan RW. Evaluation of treatment-resistant schizophrenia. *Schizophr Bull.* 1997;23:663-674.

Kane J, Honigfeld G, Singer J, Meltzer H. Clozapine for the treatment-resistant schizophrenia. A double-blind comparison with chlorpromazine. *Arch Gen Psychiatry.* 1988;45:789-796.

Kane JM. Treatment-resistant schizophrenic patients. *J Clin Psychiatry.* 1996;57(suppl 9):35-40.

Sheitman BB, Lieberman JA. The natural history and pathophysiology of treatment resistant schizophrenia. *J Psychiatr Res.* 1998; 32:143-150.

Wahlbeck K, Cheine M, Essali A, Adams C. Evidence of clozapine's effectiveness in schizophrenia: a systematic review and meta-analysis of randomized trials. *Am J Psychiatry.* 1999;156: 990-999.

Wirshing DA, Marshall BD Jr, Green MF, Mintz J, Marder SR, Wirshing WC. Risperidone in treatment-refractory schizophrenia. *Am J Psychiatry.* 1999;156:1374-1379.

9 Antipsychotics in Special Populations

Treatment of Schizophrenia in Adolescents

The diagnosis of schizophrenia in children and adolescents is often difficult to make and should be differentiated from pervasive developmental disorders, attention-deficit/hyperactivity disorder, and language or communication disorders. If a child has prominent hallucinations or delusions, however, the diagnosis of schizophrenia should be considered. Onset before the age of 18 is often classified as early-onset schizophrenia and those presenting with symptoms before the age of 14 are labeled patients with very-early-onset schizophrenia (VEOS). Although more male adolescents may develop VEOS than females (2:1), the overall prevalence is rare: 1/10,000 individuals. Auditory hallucinations are common and occur in approximately 80% of children and adolescents with schizophrenia. Command hallucinations are the most frequently occurring type of hallucination. The content and context of hallucinations in children and adolescents vary by age, with younger children tending to be less complex and less "fixed." Childhood themes, such as monsters or animals, are common but should not be mistaken for normal childhood imagination and imaginary images.

Treatment of psychotic children and adolescents ideally involves an intensive and comprehensive program. A highly structured environment with special education and psychoeducation is recommended. Day treatment, hospitalization, or long-term residential treatment may be necessary. Pharmacologic treatment is indicated if positive psychotic symptoms cause significant impairments or interfere with other interventions. Conventional antipsychotics have modest efficacy in children and adolescents (expressed in chlorpromazine [CPZ] equivalent dosages) at doses between 10 CPZ to 200 CPZ equivalents. Younger patients appear to be less responsive to pharmacotherapy than adults, however.

The low-potency agents should be avoided in this population because of sedation and cognitive dulling, which may interfere with school work. Adolescents are more vulnerable to extrapyramidal symptoms (EPS), namely dystonic reactions, than are adults. Due to concerns with EPS and tardive dyskinesia (TD) in this group, many children and adolescents are being given second-generation antipsychotic drugs (SGADs). A few open trials have reported on the use of clozapine in children and adolescents. Although most patients experience improvement during clozapine therapy, side effects in this population may be more pronounced than in adults. The most prominent symptoms seen are:

- Somnolence
- Hypersalivation
- Weight gain.

Children and adolescents tend on average to gain more weight than reported in the adult literature. Mean weight gains are over 15 pounds in 6 weeks with conventional antipsychotics. The risk for agranulocytosis appears to be similar to the risk in adults. Children and adolescents who have been found to be resistant to at least two trials of antipsychotics including another SGAD may benefit from a trial of clozapine. They should be treated initially with lower doses than adult patients and be titrated at a slower rate. Side effects should be monitored closely during initiation and throughout maintenance therapy. Enuresis may occur with clozapine therapy and often at higher rates in children and adolescents than in adults.

The use of risperidone, quetiapine, and olanzapine has also been reported in open studies and case report series. These medications appear to be similar in regard to efficacy in this population, and side effects are similar to what is observed in the adult population. Weight gain with these agents, as well, is more pronounced than in the adult population. Of these agents, olanzapine causes the greatest amount of weight gain. Prolactin-related adverse effects, especially galactorrhea, menstrual changes, and gynecomastia, occur more frequently in the younger population than in adults. Risperidone causes some of these problems more frequently than the other SGADs, but they are generally dose related.

Initial dosing for risperidone in children and adolescents should be 0.25 mg to 0.5 mg qd or bid. The range for treatment is between 0.5 mg/day and 5 mg/day. Olanzapine should be initiated at 5 mg/day and titrated to 10 mg/day to 20 mg/day. Children metabolize these drugs more rapidly than do adults but also require lower plasma levels for efficacy. Informed consent, the rationale for treatment, and potential risks and benefits of therapy should be addressed with the parents/guardians prior to treatment with any antipsychotic medication and assent should be obtained from the child. Standardized clinician ratings, such as the Positive and Negative Syndrome Scales derived from the Children's Psychiatric Rating Scale, are sensitive to antipsychotic improvement in children and adolescents.

Treatment of Psychosis in the Elderly

In the elderly, the prevalence of various types of depression, anxiety, dementia, and psychotic disorders can be as high as 50% for nursing home residents. In fact, for institutionalized patients, antipsychotics are the most widely prescribed psychotropic drugs. Because of the widespread and unnecessary use of these agents in this population in the past, Congress passed regulations for their use in 1987. This led to the introduction of Omnibus Budget Reconciliation Act and the Nursing Home Reform Amendments through the Health Care Financing Administration. These regulations set specific standards for allowable dosages and indications for psychotropic drugs in regular use and on an as-needed basis.

Antipsychotics can be safe and effective for the treatment of psychosis if used at lower doses than commonly used in young adults. Older adults are particularly vulnerable to side effects of conventional antipsychotics. Parkinsonian symptoms reportedly occur in over 50% of all elderly patients receiving these agents, and the cumulative annual incidence of TD in middle-aged and elderly patients is over 25%. The likelihood of reversing this potentially debilitating condition diminishes with age. Other adverse effects of these agents that are often intolerable in the older population include orthostatic hypotension and anticholinergic effects. Orthostasis is estimated to occur in 5% to 30% of geriatric patients and is a major contributing factor in the occurrence of falls. The elderly are more prone to consequences associated with falls, such as bone fractures, injuries, and resulting dependency. Low-potency agents and clozapine are more likely to cause significant drops in orthostatic blood pressure. Anticholinergic effects in the elderly may cause such side effects as:

- Constipation
- Dry mouth
- Urinary retention
- Cognitive impairment.

The elderly are especially sensitive to these effects, and the use of laxatives or stool softeners is particularly high in nursing homes. Cognitive impairment may lead to decreased independence, and a more rapid decline in cognitive functioning may occur in elderly patients treated with antipsychotics than in the younger adult population.

Clozapine has been used successfully in the elderly population at lower doses than in younger adult patients. Mean doses have ranged from 50 mg/day to 300 mg/day, with a much slower rate of titration. Clozapine may be a good selection for treating psychotic elderly patients with preexisting parkinsonism because of this drug's lower affinity for dopamine $(D)_2$ receptors in the striatum. Clinically, however, it is a poorly tolerated antipsychotic in geriatric patients and should be used with caution. The risk for agranulocytosis appears to be about 4% in the elderly population, with older women being at highest risk. The risk for seizure activity is increased in the elderly, and sedation is one of the major reasons for discontinuation. Clozapine therapy should be initiated at 12.5 mg/day to 25 mg/day given in two divided doses, titrating by increments of 12.5 mg over 5 to 7 days. 9

Risperidone has been shown to be effective in the elderly with schizophrenia, schizoaffective disorder, major depression with psychotic features, bipolar disorder, and delusional disorder. A dose range of 0.5 mg to 3 mg is the optimal range for the treatment of psychotic symptoms in the elderly. Initially, patients should receive 0.25 mg to 0.5 mg taken once daily, with titration in increments not greater than 0.5 mg/24 hours. In most studies, risperidone is well tolerated, with the most common side effects being hypotension, orthostasis, sedation, and EPS. Olanzapine and quetiapine have been reported to be of benefit in the elderly population, but no results of large-scale controlled studies are yet available. A starting dose of olanzapine should be 2.5 mg/day to 10 mg/day and increased by 5 mg no more frequently than every 7 days to a target range of 10 mg/day to 20 mg/day. Lower doses of quetiapine should be used as well. These agents appear to have adverse-effect profiles similar to those in the adult population.

Treatment of Schizophrenia in Dually Diagnosed Patients

The prevalence of substance abuse among persons with schizophrenia is significantly higher than in the general population. Conservative estimates are that one third to as many as one half of people with schizophrenia abuse alcohol and illicit drugs. Dually diagnosed patients are more likely to be noncompliant with treatment and medications often because of side effects. These people also have a poorer response rate to conventional antipsychotics and have higher rates of rehospitalization. For patients discharged on conventional antipsychotics, substance abuse is one of the most significant reasons for readmission. EPS may occur more frequently in patients who are substance abusing, and abusing drugs and alcohol is a risk factor for developing TD.

There is evidence that substance-abusing patients respond differently to conventional antipsychotics compared with non–substance-abusing patients. A few studies have reported that substance-abusing patients receiving fixed doses of haloperidol and perphenazine had a poorer response and more readmissions than non–substance-abusing patients. This is likely due to the fact that substance abusers suffer increased rates of parkinsonian side effects from conventional antipsychotics and are less compliant than nonabusing patients. Substance abuse itself can lead to chronic psychosis and psychotic relapse. Despite the fact that substance-abusing patients do poorly with conventional antipsychotic treatment, this group has been found to have better premorbid functioning and less functional impairment than non–substance-abusing schizophrenic patients. It is possible that while patients in this group are difficult to treat, they may also present a subgroup with a better potential for recovery and perhaps a better opportunity for successful reintegration into community living.

Second-generation antipsychotic drugs may offer effective clinical treatment for schizophrenic patients involved in comorbid substance abuse. It has been reported that treatment with clozapine and olanzapine is associated with similar response rates between patients with and without substance abuse histories. Additionally, these medications are associated with better compliance rates than conventional agents, as well as lower rates of rehospitalization. Further evidence indicates that clozapine treatment may actually be associated with a reduction in the use of drugs and alcohol. Case reports of patients treated with risperidone who are substance abusers report that it not only is efficacious for symptoms but may help curb use as well. Thus substance-abusing patients may benefit from SGADs in terms of both better efficacy and adverse-effect profiles.

Treatment of Schizophrenia With Mood and Anxiety Symptoms

When Kraepelin first described psychosis, he divided symptoms into dementia praecox and manic-depressive psychosis. This division failed, however, to include many patients with mixed features. Approximately 30% to 60% of patients with schizophrenia report an episode of major depression at some point in their lifetime. Schizoaffective disorder or schizophrenia with concurrent depression is an example of patients with primary psychosis in conjunction with prominent mood symptoms. Although mood stabilizers and antidepressants are ineffective for psychosis, they may offer benefits to patients for relief of symptoms associated with mood. It is important to remember that as other medications are added to the regimen, specific target symptoms should be identified and objective rating criteria should be utilized to assess efficacy.

Second-generation antipsychotic drugs may be effective as monotherapy for schizoaffective disorder. Clozapine has been found to be more effective in patients with schizoaffective disorder than in those with schizophrenia. Schizoaffective disorder, in fact, has been found to be a predictor of clozapine response in treatment-resistant populations. There is accumulating evidence that risperidone, olanzapine, and quetiapine all may be beneficial for schizoaffective disorder as well as bipolar disorder. This evidence suggests that SGADs are more effective than conventional antipsychotics for mood symptoms. Monotherapy should be attempted in these disorders prior to polytherapy.

Anticonvulsants and mood stabilizers in combination with antipsychotics have been more effective for schizoaffective disorder than antipsychotics plus placebo. This has not been found to be true, however, for patients with schizophrenia lacking a mood component. Lithium, valproate, and carbamazepine appear to offer benefits, but few large well-controlled studies have looked at treatment specifically for schizoaffective disorder. Carbamazepine is a potent inducer of the cytochrome P450 (CYP450) 3A3/4 pathway, thus it potentially may lower blood levels of quetiapine. Carbamazepine should not be used concurrently with clozapine due to the risk for the occurrence of agranulocytosis. Lithium may increase leukocytes, thus has the potential to mask neutropenia with clozapine treatment. Valproate may increase plasma levels of clozapine or olanzapine through inhibition of CYP450 2D6. This is not a potent effect of valproate, but a few patients will experience an increase in plasma concentrations. Valproate and lithium also increase the risk for weight gain with antipsychotic treatment.

Little work has been done in looking at antidepressant use in combination with antipsychotics for the treatment of schizoaffective disorder or schizophrenia with depression. The most widely accepted data for patient depression with schizophrenia or schizoaffective disorder concern the treatment of depressive symptoms after stabilization of psychosis. If antidepressants are concurrently used, the possibility for drug interaction exists. Fluvoxamine, a potent inhibitor of the CYP450 1A2 isoenzyme, will increase blood levels of clozapine and olanzapine. Fluoxetine, paroxetine, and higher doses of sertraline may increase blood levels as well. SGADs, although not studied in monotherapy for depression, appear to intrinsically offer some benefits for affective symptoms such as anxiety and depression. 9

Patients who continue to exhibit significant symptoms of anxiety once stabilization of psychosis is accomplished may benefit from anxiolytic therapy. The concurrent use of benzodiazepines and clozapine should be avoided, if possible, due to the increased risk for sudden respiratory depression that may occur with the combination. Also, benzodiazepines may lead to cognitive dulling or paradoxic agitation. Thus, in patients with deficits in cognitive functioning intrinsic to schizophrenia itself, the use of another contributing agent should be strongly evaluated. Buspirone may work for anxiety but may be less effective in patients who have already received benzodiazepine therapy.

SUGGESTED READING

Buckley PF. Substance abuse in schizophrenia: a review. *J Clin Psychiatry*. 1998;59(suppl 3):26-30.

Campbell M, Rapoport JL, Simpson GM. Antipsychotics in children and adolescents. *J Am Acad Child Adolesc Psychiatry*. 1999; 38:537-545.

Collaborative Working Group on Clinical Trial Evaluations. Treatment of special populations with the atypical antipsychotics. *J Clin Psychiatry*. 1998;59(suppl 12):46-52.

Findling RL, Schulz SC, Reed MD, Blumer JL. The antipsychotics. A pediatric perspective. *Pediatr Clin North Am*. 1998;45: 1205-1232.

Jeste DV, Rockwell E, Harris MJ, Lohr JB, Lacro J. Conventional vs. newer antipsychotics in elderly patients. *Am J Geriatr Psychiatry*. 1999;7:70-76.

Krystal JH, D'Souza DC, Madonick S, Petrakis IL. Toward a rational pharmacotherapy of comorbid substance abuse in schizophrenic patients. *Schizophr Res*. 1999;35(suppl):S35-S49.

Levinson DF, Umapathy C, Musthaq M. Treatment of schizoaffective disorder and schizophrenia with mood symptoms. *Am J Psychiatry*. 1999;156:1138-1148.

Maixner SM, Mellow AM, Tandon R. The efficacy, safety, and tolerability of antipsychotics in the elderly. *J Clin Psychiatry*. 1999;60(suppl 8):29-41.

McClellan J, Werry JS. Practice parameters for the assessment and treatment of children and adolescents with schizophrenia. American Academy of Child and Adolescent Psychiatry. *J Am Acad Child Adolesc Psychiatry*. 1997;36(suppl 10):177S-193S.

Toren P, Laor N, Weizman A. Use of atypical neuroleptics in child and adolescent psychiatry. *J Clin Psychiatry*. 1998;59:644-656.

10 Drug Interactions With Antipsychotics

Pharmacokinetics is the study of how the body acts upon drugs, especially in terms of absorption, distribution, metabolism, and excretion. Interactions may occur during any of these processes as a drug is transported to and from its site of action and may result in a change in the plasma level or tissue distribution of the drug. Pharmacodynamics refers to the effect of the drugs on the body. This type of interaction occurs at biologically active receptor sites and results in a change in the pharmacologic effects of a given plasma level of the drug. This chapter will focus mainly on pharmacokinetic drug interactions.

Absorption

Gastrointestinal drug absorption can be altered by the concomitant administration of a second drug, food product, herbal supplement, or an environmental product that physically or chemically binds to the drug, increases or decreases gut motility, alters intestinal bacterial flora, or changes gastric pH. Antacids, charcoal, and cholestyramine are agents that can bind to other agents and form insoluble complexes. Antacids should always be given 2 hours apart from antipsychotics to avoid decreasing absorption. Most of the antipsychotics are not affected by food. Absorption of quetiapine, however, may be increased with meals. In addition, the antipsychotic solutions should not be given with other solutions (such as carbamazepine and lithium) as insoluble complexes may form.

Distribution

In general, the antipsychotics have a relatively high affinity for plasma proteins, with most being greater than 80% protein bound. A reversible equilibrium exists between bound and unbound drug; the unbound fraction is pharmacologically active, whereas the bound fraction is inactive and cannot be metabolized or excreted. When two drugs exist simultaneously in the plasma, competition for protein-binding sites may occur. This may result in the displacement of a previously bound drug, which, in the free state, becomes pharmacologically active. Interactions that occur by this mechanism are called "protein-binding interactions." Most protein-binding interactions are transient and are not clinically significant because the plasma concentration change of free drug is generally quite small. Clinically significant interactions may occur with antipsychotics when given with another highly protein-bound drug with a low therapeutic index such as warfarin or phenytoin.

Metabolism

All antipsychotic agents are metabolized by hepatic microsomal enzymes to water-soluble compounds that can be excreted by the kidneys. The most important of the microsomal enzymes are the cytochrome P450 (CYP450) enzymes, a group of nonspecific mixed-function oxidases that play a major role in oxidative drug metabolism. Although more than 30 isoenzymes have been identified in humans, three play major roles in the metabolism of antipsychotic medications:

- CYP450 2D6
- CYP450 1A2
- CYP450 3A3/4.

Not all individuals have the same CYP450 enzymes. If mutations occur in more than 1% of a specific population, it is termed pharmacogenetic polymorphism. For example, about 5% to 10% of Caucasians are poor metabolizers via the CYP450 2D6 enzyme. Thus these people must metabolize drugs by alternative routes that may not be as efficient as the 2D6 route, leading to increases in plasma concentrations for the drug to be metabolized. The major enzymes for metabolism of second-generation antipsychotic drugs (SGADs) and a few known for traditional antipsychotics are listed in Table 10.1.

Other medications, food products, herbal supplements, and environmental factors may inhibit or induce any of these pathways, possibly lowering or raising plasma concentrations of any of the antipsychotic medications. Table 10.2 provides a list of some substances that may affect metabolism.

A listing of likely interactions with SGADs that may be clinically significant appears in Table 10.3.

TABLE 10.1 — MAJOR ENZYMES FOR METABOLISM OF ANTIPSYCHOTIC DRUGS

Drug	Major Metabolic Pathway	Other Metabolic Pathways
Clozapine	1A2	3A3/4, 2D6
Haloperidol	2D6	—
Olanzapine	1A2	2D6
Perphenazine	2D6	—
Quetiapine	3A3/4	—
Risperidone	2D6	—
Thioridazine	2D6	—
Ziprasidone*	3A3/4	—

* Investigational.

TABLE 10.2 — SUBSTANCES THAT MAY AFFECT METABOLISM OF ANTIPSYCHOTIC DRUGS

Type of Agent	CYP450 1A2	CYP450 2D6	CYP450 3A3/4
Inducing agents	Cigarette smoking Omeprazole	—	Carbamazepine Phenytoin Phenobarbital Rifampin
Inhibiting agents	Fluvoxamine Fluoxetine (weak) Fluoroquinolines Cimetidine	Fluoxetine Paroxetine Sertraline (weak, dose-related) Tertiary tricyclic antidepressants Haloperidol (weak) Thioridazine (weak) Perphenazine (weak) Quinidine	Fluoxetine Nefazadone Ketoconazole Itraconazole Erythromycin Protease inhibitors Cisapride Verapamil Diltiazem Grapefruit

Abbreviations: CYP450, cytochrome P450.

TABLE 10.3 — CLINICALLY IMPORTANT INTERACTIONS WITH SECOND-GENERATION ANTIPSYCHOTIC DRUGS

Drug	Drug Interaction
Clozapine	Inhibitors of cytochrome P450 (CYP450) 1A2 (fluvoxamine, others) can raise clozapine levels. Cigarette smoking can decrease clozapine level; watch for relapse if patient begins or increases smoking. Inhibitors of CYP450 2D6 can raise clozapine levels. Strong inhibitors of CYP450 3A3/4 can raise clozapine levels.
Olanzapine	Inhibitors of CYP450 1A2 can raise olanzapine levels. Cigarette smoking can decrease olanzapine levels. Inhibitors of CYP450 2D6 may raise olanzapine levels. Women have higher plasma concentrations than men; may need lower doses.
Ziprasidone*	Strong inhibitors of CYP450 3A3/4 may raise ziprasidone levels.

* Investigational.

Clinically meaningful interactions with risperidone and quetiapine are unlikely. Clozapine and olanzapine may be affected by other substances, and high blood levels of ziprasidone may theoretically lead to possible prolongations of the QT interval.

Excretion

The kidney is the major organ for drug excretion. Renal excretion of active drug can be altered by the concurrent administration of any drug that affects renal blood flow, active tubular secretion, or passive tubular reabsorption. These types of interactions with antipsychotics are uncommon. Lithium is one psychotropic that is highly affected by other medications altering these parameters.

SUGGESTED READING

Fang J, Gorrod JW. Metabolism, pharmacogenetics, and metabolic drug-drug interactions of antipsychotic drugs. *Cell Mol Neurobiol.* 1999;19:491-510.

Jefferson JW. Drug interactions—friend or foe? *J Clin Psychiatry.* 1998;59(suppl 4):37-47.

Ketter TA, Flockhart DA, Post RM, et al. The emerging role of cytochrome P450 3A in psychopharmacology. *J Clin Psychopharmacol.* 1995;15:387-398.

Maixner SM, Mellow AM, Tandon R. The efficacy, safety, and tolerability of antipsychotics in the elderly. *J Clin Psychiatry.* 1999; 60(suppl 8):29-41.

Shen WW. The metabolism of atypical antipsychotic drugs: an update. *Ann Clin Psychiatry.* 1999;11:145-158.

Tanaka E, Hisawa S. Clinically significant pharmacokinetic drug interactions with psychoactive drugs: antidepressants and antipsychotics and the cytochrome P450 system. *J Clin Pharm Ther.* 1999;24:7-16.

11 Cognition and Antipsychotics

It is estimated that approximately 40% of patients with schizophrenia have impairments in neurocognition. These deficits in cognition are thought to be the result of abnormalities in the frontal and temporal lobes and/or altered connectivity between these regions. The major deficits in patients with schizophrenia are:

- Executive function (abstraction/flexibility)
- Attention
- Verbal fluency
- Learning and memory
- Spatial and verbal working memory
- Semantic memory
- Psychomotor performance.

Functional consequences of these deficits have been found to be clinically relevant. Quality-of-life measures have been highly correlated with cognitive impairment. Executive functioning is related to community functioning, and verbal memory is associated with community function, social problem solving, and skill acquisition. Occupational and social dysfunction are present in most people with schizophrenia. Cognitive deficits prevent many patients with schizophrenia from functioning socially and maintaining employment.

Traditional Antipsychotics

There is no consistent evidence that traditional antipsychotics have positive effects on cognition. Low-potency antipsychotics, such as thioridazine, chlorpromazine, and mesoridazine, may actually worsen working memory, likely due to anticholinergic effects. In fact, cognition has been found to improve in patients once thioridazine is discontinued. Extrapyramidal symptoms (EPS) may also affect motor tasks where speed and accuracy are required. Haloperidol was found to impair higher cognitive functions such as ability to assess one's performance and to shift strategies. Small positive effects have been noted, primarily in attention and semantic memory. Beneficial effects of traditional antipsychotics usually appear only after prolonged treatment and are mainly in sustained attention and visuomotor tasks. Negative effects that occur with acute and chronic treatment with conventional antipsychotics are primarily deficits in attention vigilance and motor skills.

Second-Generation Antipsychotic Drugs

Clozapine has shown some benefits on verbal fluency, semantic memory, attention, and some types of executive functioning. Clozapine has been reported to cause negative results on working memory, possibly due to its dopamine $(D)_1$ antagonist properties, anticholinergic effects, or sedating effects. Risperidone seems to produce different results than those produced by clozapine; patients with schizophrenia who take risperidone have shown improvement in working memory. Risperidone has been shown to improve selective attention, reaction time, alertness, and motor coordination. These effects are possibly due to 5-hydroxytryptamine $(5\text{-HT})_{2A}$ receptor antagonism, the lower rates of EPS, the lower affinity for cholinergic receptors, and the lack of sedation. Treatment with olanzapine has shown improvement in attention, executive functioning, motor skills, learning and memory, and spatial ability. Preliminary data report that quetiapine treatment is associated with improvement in attention and learning. Although cognitive benefits of these drugs look promising, much work is needed in this area to ascertain the specific cognitive benefits of the second-generation antipsychotic drugs.

Glutaminergic transmission is known to play a fundamental role in cognitive processes. Accumulating evidence suggests that reduced excitatory glutaminergic activity could underlie some symptoms of the disease. Imaging and postmortem studies in patients with schizophrenia have revealed abnormalities in a number of brain regions that are connected by glutamateric circuits. Furthermore, noncompetitive antagonists of *N*-methyl-D-aspartate (NMDA) receptors, such as phencyclidine and ketamine, exacerbate or produce symptoms and may temporarily decrease cognitive functioning. A family of drugs, the ampakines, enhance excitatory (glutaminergic) transmission and enhance learning and memory in rodents, suggesting this group of drugs may improve cognitive dysfunction in patients. CX516 (Ampalex) is in phase II clinical trials and may be promising for improvements in this symptom domain. In a small sample of patients on clozapine, CX516 (Ampalex) improved memory and attention on a number of neuropsychiatric tests. This drug may also be beneficial in patients with Alzheimer's disease.

SUGGESTED READING

Collaborative Working Group on Clinical Trial Evaluations. Evaluating the effects of antipsychotics on cognition in schizophrenia. *J Clin Psychiatry*. 1998;59(suppl 12):35-40.

Goldberg TE, Weinberger DR. Effects of neuroleptic medications on the cognition of patients with schizophrenia: a review of recent studies. *J Clin Psychiatry*. 1996;57(suppl 9):62-65.

Green MF, Nuechterlein KH. Should schizophrenia be treated as a neurocognitive disorder? *Schizophr Bull*. 1999;25:309-319.

Jeste DV, Lohr JB, Eastham JH, Rockwell E, Caligiuri MP. Adverse neurobiological effects of long-term use of neuroleptics: human and animal studies. *J Psychiatr Res*. 1998;32:201-214.

Meltzer HY, McGurk SR. The effects of clozapine, risperidone, and olanzapine on cognitive function in schizophrenia. *Schizophr Bull*. 1999;25:233-255.

Rund BR, Borg NE. Cognitive deficits and cognitive training in schizophrenic patients: a review. *Acta Psychiatr Scand*. 1999;100: 85-95.

12 Outcomes and Health-Services Research

Long-term outcomes for many people with schizophrenia remain disappointing. Approximately 10% of people with schizophrenia are at risk for suicide and fewer than 20% will be employed in competitive work at any time. Preventing relapse is critical to improving all areas of long-term outcome. Without effective maintenance therapy and with the occurrence of high relapse rates, improving patient functioning and quality of life will not be accomplished.

Relapse and Rehospitalization

Up to one half of all stabilized patients may be readmitted within 1 year following discharge. It is known that the more relapses and periods off medication, the poorer the prognosis and long-term outcome for schizophrenic patients. Medication noncompliance is one of the more significant factors leading to relapse in schizophrenia. In the outpatient setting, noncompliance rates in patients with schizophrenia are as high as 50%. This may be due to:

- Illness-related issues, such as lack of insight
- Treatment management issues, such as inadequate support
- Drug-related issues, such as intolerable side effects.

Extrapyramidal symptoms (EPS), including dystonic reactions, akathisia, and persistent pseudoparkinsonism, may explain why some patients stop taking antipsychotic medications once discharged from the hospital. Second-generation antipsychotic drugs (SGADs), such as clozapine, risperidone, olanzapine, and quetiapine, are associated with much better side effect profiles as compared with conventional agents. Thus SGADs theoretically may increase patient compliance due to a better risk-benefit profile with respect to clinical efficacy and adverse effects.

Treatment with conventional antipsychotics has been found to be associated with 1-year recidivism rates around 40% to 50%; however, these rates may be decreased with the combination of depot neuroleptic use and intense therapy. Fluphenazine decanoate in combination with social therapy may lower relapse rates to around 23% per year. Fluphenazine decanoate therapy in combination with intense applied family management was associated with a 26% rehospitalization rate over a 2-year period. Although these results are much improved under optimal conditions, the actual "real-world use" of treatment with therapeutic doses of depot medications is probably associated with a higher rate of recidivism.

There is good evidence that the SGADs are more protective against relapse than are the conventional antipsychotics. One-year rehospitalization rates of treatment-resistant patients receiving clozapine are between 13% and 18% per year. Rehospitalization rates for risperidone, olanzapine, and quetiapine are approximately 12% to 19%. These medications have all been shown to decrease the length of hospital stays as well. Because hospital stays are the primary determinants of overall costs, SGADs can be cost-effective if they are associated with lower rates of rehospitalization.

Quality of Life and Employment

The symptoms and cognitive disturbances of schizophrenia lead to great disability in social and work functioning. Less than 20% of all patients with schizophrenia are employed. In the past, treatment focused on immediate symptom relief, while issues relating to quality of life were largely neglected. Quality of life refers to a patient's subjective sense of well-being. The concept may include:

- Social issues
- Economic well-being
- Fulfillment of personal aspirations
- Relationships.

Other medical or medication issues, such as medication side effects, can relate strongly to the perceived sense of well-being.

The psychiatric field has begun to recognize the importance of these issues in the treatment of schizophrenia. Conventional antipsychotics have produced cognitive and affective impairments influencing well-being, as well as EPS, sexual dysfunction, and tardive dyskinesia, which further lead to a sense of poor quality of life. There is growing evidence that people treated with SGADs compared with conventional agents have a significantly higher general quality of life. This has been reported in long-term treatment with clozapine, olanzapine, risperidone, and quetiapine compared with conventional antipsychotics.

Economics of Schizophrenia

While safety and efficacy of a particular treatment are the primary considerations in selecting an antipsychotic medication, other costs are important to consider as well. The treatment of schizophrenia alone accounts for about 2.5% of the total health-care expenditures nationally, with over $32.5 billion being spent in the United States annually. SGADs compared with the conventional agents offer many benefits to treatment, although the higher pricing of SGADs represents a deterrent to their routine use.

Economic analysis techniques are becoming more rigorous and sophisticated as pharmacoeconomic issues are increasingly important in the decision-making process for service providers. There are four principle ways or carrying out economic evaluations as listed in Table 12.1.

The gold standard for cost-effectiveness analysis is the medical-effectiveness study, a prospective randomized trial designed primarily to obtain cost-effectiveness information. These data can also be obtained by collecting cost data during the typical double-blind, randomized, controlled efficacy trial. Retrospective studies are generally easier to conduct but may be more difficult to interpret. Most published studies involving any of the SGADs and costs are retrospective and/or naturalistic in nature. Although there is little standardization of the variables and methods included in the cost equations, there is consistency in reporting that SGADs are actually more cost-effective or cost-beneficial compared with conventional antipsychotics when total care is measured.

A large prospective comparative trial found clozapine to be superior to haloperidol while costing over $2000 less per patient per year in overall costs. Several other retrospective studies found that treatment with clozapine decreased overall costs per patient per year as compared with prior therapy. Pharmacoeconomic research with risperidone has reported a decrease in hospital stays as compared with conventional antipsychotic therapy. Studies have reported an average savings of between $1000 and $5000 per patient per year, and similar results have been seen with

TABLE 12.1 — ECONOMIC EVALUATIONS OF SCHIZOPHRENIA	
Analysis Method	**Process**
Cost minimization	This process evaluates the costs of alternative treatment methods. The usual assumption in these studies is that two alternative treatments produce identical outcomes and therefore the least costly method is preferred.
Cost benefit	This analysis compares two treatment approaches and estimates in purely monetary terms the costs and benefits of alternatives. The studies do not include personal costs and benefits since these costs are impossible to value in monetary terms in a realistic way.
Cost-effectiveness	In this analysis, costs are estimated for achieving outcomes such as life-years gained, years of work restored, or time without positive symptoms of schizophrenia.
Cost utility	This analysis requires valid and easily used quality-of-life measures. These results can be combined with survival data to produce estimates of quality-adjusted life-years.

olanzapine. Little work has been done with quetiapine, and ziprasidone has not yet been marketed. These, too, may prove to be beneficial for cost savings. There are few data with which to compare the costs among the SGADs. Because all of the drugs appear to decrease the rate of rehospitalization as well as the length of hospital stays, the main differences in costs would be in the use of outpatient services and the drug costs themselves. The cost of risperidone and quetiapine, for the average doses utilized, is approximately one half that of olanzapine and clozapine. Large prospective controlled trials are needed to ascertain specific differences in overall costs among the SGADs.

SUGGESTED READING

Browne S, Garavan J, Gervin M, Roe M, Larkin C, O'Callaghan E. Quality of life in schizophrenia: insight and subjective response to neuroleptics. *J Nerv Ment Dis*. 1998;186:74-78.

Fleischhacker WW, Hummer M. Drug treatment of schizophrenia in the 1990s. Achievements and future possibilities in optimising outcomes. *Drugs*. 1997;53:915-929.

Franz M, Lis S, Pluddemann K, Gallhofer B. Conventional versus atypical neuroleptics: subjective quality of life in schizophrenic patients. *Br J Psychiatry*. 1997;170:422-425.

Lauriello J, Bustillo J, Keith SJ. A critical review of research on psychosocial treatment of schizophrenia. *Biol Psychiatry*. 1999;46:1409-1417.

Lehman AF. Developing an outcomes-oriented approach for the treatment of schizophrenia. *J Clin Psychiatry*. 1999;60(suppl 19):30-35; discussion 36-37.

Weiden P, Aquila R, Standard J. Atypical antipsychotic drugs and long-term outcome in schizophrenia. *J Clin Psychiatry*. 1996;57(suppl 11):53-60.

Williams R, Dickson RA. Economics of schizophrenia. *Can J Psychiatry*. 1995;40(suppl 2):S60-S67.

13 Future Directions

We have begun a paradigm shift in the pharmacologic treatment of psychoses. Second-generation antipsychotic drugs (SGADs) are replacing the conventional agents that have been the mainstay of treatment for almost 40 years. While the dopamine theory of psychosis has been tremendously useful in understanding and modeling this disorder, we now know that SGADs may work through other mechanisms of action. Besides being effective for positive and negative symptoms, when compared with conventional agents, SGADs:

- Cause fewer side effects
- Lessen cognitive impairment
- Lead to a better quality of life
- Have antidepressant effects
- Have much lower relapse and rehospitalization rates.

Because of their improved tolerability and outcomes, these drugs hold more promise in patients with affective components, comorbid substance-abuse histories, and young and elderly patients. Thus, one important direction for future research would be to better study current SGADs in subpopulations with schizophrenia.

A second important direction for research is to further address and characterize the limitations and differences among the current compounds. Issues such as weight gain, elevated prolactin levels, and the impact on long-term morbidity and mortality should be addressed. The use of antipsychotics in the treatment of acutely agitated or aggressive patients and better characterization of dosing are other important areas for future research.

New formulations of currently marketed compounds may provide increased ease and compliance with use. Risperidone, olanzapine, and ziprasidone are all under study for the depot formulations. Quetiapine is being studied in long-acting tablets to allow for less-frequent dosing. Risperidone is available currently as an oral solution and olanzapine will soon be available as a sublingual, rapidly dissolving wafer. Combination agents, such as a fluoxetine/olanzapine product, are also being studied.

Several new products are under investigation in phase II and III studies. Zotepine and MDL 100,907 were two up-and-coming agents which had differing properties, the inhibition of norepinephrine reuptake and selective 5-hydroxytryptamine $(5\text{-HT})_{2A}$ antagonism, respectively. These two compounds, however, were recently pulled from trials in US markets. Iloperidone (Zomaril) is currently in phase III trials, including a large multinational trial of over 3000 patients. This agent has a high 5-HT–to–dopamine $(D)_2$ affinity and appears to be effective for positive and negative symptoms. It has a receptor-binding profile similar to that of risperidone. The half-life is about 13 hours to 14 hours and the most common adverse effects are orthostasis, dizziness, and somnolence. Aripiprazole has recently entered phase III trials. This agent is a potent D_2 antagonist but also is a presynaptic D_2 agonist causing it to have few extrapyramidal symptoms. The half-life of this agent is 46 hours, which may aid in new dosing strategies. CX516 (Ampalex), which may augment antipsychotics for neurocognition (see Chapter 11, *Cognition and Antipsychotics*) is in phase II trials, as is PNU 101387, a D_4 antagonist. Preclinical data hint that other emerging compounds may work by other mechanisms such as inhibiting sigma receptors (SR-31742), modifications of glutamate or nicotine, and inhibition of fatty-acid breakdown (SC-111).

As we consider these exciting new medications, we need to keep in mind the continuing limitations of currently marketed drugs and the sparsity of new agents in the next several years. We must be aware that new, effective therapies for schizophrenia will unlikely be simple in their clinical use. As the psychiatric field works to more accurately identify people who are vulnerable to psychosis and to understand brain regions associated with this illness, we should work to more effectively integrate current treatment options with active psychosocial and rehabilitative programming to attempt to provide beneficial treatment for the people we see today. People who suffer from schizophrenia today will benefit from optimized medication therapy. These benefits include marked improvements in functioning and quality of life.

The pharmacotherapy of schizophrenia has evolved from a relatively simple strategy, involving a homogeneous class of medications with a high ratio of behavioral toxicity to beneficial effects to a more complex group of drugs with improved efficacy. There is, however, no magic bullet or correct therapy for all patients. Clinicians should now attempt to optimize therapy for each patient in a highly individualized way.

INDEX

Note: Page numbers in *italics* indicate figures;
page numbers followed by t indicate tables.

14

14

14

14

14

14